Praise for
Mental Health Survival Kit and Withdrawal from Psychiatric Drugs

"Peter Gøtzsche's new book meets patients' need to get tools on how to deal with psychoactive drugs and, above all, not to start them. Gøtzsche is very clear about the role of GPs in medicalizing grief, misfortune, opposition, and bad luck. In this he finds the American emeritus professor of psychiatry and chairman of the DSM-III committee, Allen Frances, at his side. Both Gøtzsche and Frances have repeatedly stated that psychoactive drugs should not be prescribed by GPs because they lack experience in their use. And above all, unhappiness, grief, and bad luck are not signs of brain disorders, they belong to daily life." Additionally, Gøtzsche reveals that most psychoactive drugs do not work—'they might only achieve statistically significant differences compared to placebo, but that's not what patients need.'"

—Dick Bijl, former GP, epidemiologist, and current president of the International Society of Drug Bulletins.

"Peter C. Gøtzsche wrote this book to help people with mental health problems survive and return to a normal life. His book explains in detail how psychiatric drugs are harmful and people are told how they can safely withdraw from them. It also advises on how people with mental health problems can avoid making a 'career' as a psychiatric patient and losing 10 or 15 years of their life to psychiatry. You will find precious material to help plan and accompany this process of liberation from psychiatry."

—Fernando Freitas, PhD, Psychologist, Full Professor and Researcher at the National School of Public Health (ENSP/FIOCRUZ). Co-editor of *Mad in Brazil*

Mental Health Survival Kit and Withdrawal from Psychiatric Drugs:

A User's Guide

Peter C. Gøtzsche

Institute for Scientific Freedom

Copenhagen, Denmark

Mental Health Survival Kit and Withdrawal from Psychiatric Drugs: A User's Guide

ISBN 978-1-61599-619-3 paperback
ISBN 978-1-61599-620-9 hardcover
ISBN 978-1-61599-621-6 eBook

Institute for Scientific Freedom
Copenhagen, Denmark
www.scientificfreedom.dk
pcg@scientificfreedom.dk

Published by
L H Press, Inc.   www.LHPress.com
5145 Pontiac Trail   info@LHPress.com
Ann Arbor, MI 48105

Tollfree 888-761-6268 (USA/Canada)
Fax 734-663-6861

Distributed by Ingram (USA/CAN/AU), Bertram's Books (UK/EU)

Contents

Index of Tables and Figures

Acknowledgements

I am grateful for the thousands of emails I have received from patients and relatives describing the harms and abuses they have experienced in psychiatry and for the many interactions I have had with inspiring psychiatrists, psychologists, pharmacists and other professsionals, including Peter Breggin, Jane Bækgaard, James Davies, Magnus Hald, David Healy, Göran Högberg, Niall McLaren, Joanna Moncrieff, Luke Montagu, Klaus Munkholm, Peer Nielsen, Åsa Nilsonne, John Read, Bertel Rüdinger, Olga Runciman, Kristian Sloth, Anders Sørensen, Sami Timimi, Birgit Toft and Robert Whitaker.

Abbreviations

DSM: Diagnostic and Statistical Manual of Mental Disorders
EMA: European Medicines Agency
FDA: US Food and Drug Administration
SSRI: Selective Serotonin Reuptake Inhibitor
WHO: World Health Organization

1   This Book Might Save Your Life

I have written this book to help patients, and when I decided to write it, one of my tentative titles was, "Listening to the voices of patients." Most people I have talked to about mental health issues, be it my family, friends, colleagues, sports partners, filmmakers, gardeners, cleaners, waiters and hotel receptionists, have had bad experiences with psychiatry or know someone that have.

Coming from a background of being a specialist in internal medicine, which is entirely different, it slowly dawned on me how harmful psychiatry is. It takes years of close study to find out that psychiatry does vastly more harm than good,[1] and my own research has contributed to revealing this.

My findings resonate closely with what the general public have concluded based on their own experiences. A survey of 2,031 Australians showed that people thought that depression pills (usually called antidepressants), psychosis pills (usually called antipsychotics), electroshock and admission to a psychiatric ward were more often harmful than beneficial.[2] The social psychiatrists who had done the survey were dissatisfied with the answers and argued that people should be trained to arrive at the "right opinion."

In early 1992, the UK Royal College of Psychiatrists, in association with the Royal College of General Practitioners, launched a five-year "Defeat Depression Campaign."[3] Its aim was to provide public education about depression and its treatment in order to encourage earlier treatment-seeking and reduce stigma. Campaign activities included newspaper and magazine articles, television and radio interviews, press conferences, production of leaflets, factsheets in ethnic minority languages, audio cassettes, a self-help video and two books.[4] When 2,003 lay people were surveyed just before the launch of the campaign, 91% thought that people with depression should be offered counselling; only 16% thought they should be offered depression pills; only 46% said they were effective; and 78% regarded them as addictive.[3] The psychiatrists' view on these responses was that, "Doctors have an important role in educating the public about depression and the rationale for antidepressant treatment. In particular, patients should know that dependence is not a problem with antidepressants."

When challenged about the fact that the colleges had accepted donations from all the major manufacturers of depression pills for the campaign, the president of the Royal College of Psychiatrists, Robert Kendall, acknowledged that, "One of their major motives was the hope that an increased recognition of depressive illnesses both by the general public and by general practitioners would result in increased sales for them."[5] He didn't say what the companies' other major motives were. I doubt there were any. Money is the only motive drug companies have.

The psychiatrists embarked on their re-education campaign. But people were not easily convinced that they were wrong. A 1998 paper reported that changes were of the order of only 5-10% and that depression pills were still being regarded as addictive and less effective than counselling.[4] Interestingly, 81% of the lay people agreed that, "Depression is a medical condition like other illnesses" and 43% ascribed depression to biological changes in the brain, but most people nonetheless ascribed it to social causes like bereavement (83%), unemployment (83%), financial problems (82%), stress (83%), loneliness/ isolation (79%) and divorce/ end of relationship (83%).[4] Something didn't add up.

My interpretation is that despite claims through many years, also long before 1992,[1] that psychiatric disorders are caused by chemical imbalances in the brain, the public is not so willing to accept this falsehood.

In 2005, Danish psychiatrists reported what 493 patients had told them about their depression pill treatment.[6] About half the patients agreed that the treatment could alter their personality and that they had less control over their thoughts and feelings. Four-fifths agreed that as long as they took the drugs, they didn't really know if they were necessary, and 56% agreed to the statement that, "Your body can become addicted to antidepressants." The psychiatrists refused flatly to believe what the patients had told them, which they considered wrong, and they called them ignorant. They also felt that the patients needed "psychoeducation." The problem with this was that the relatives shared the patients' opinion.

"Educating the public" and "psychoeducation" so that they can arrive at the "right opinion" is what we normally call brainwashing. Particularly when what the patients and the public reported are more than just opinions; they drew conclusions based on their own experience and that of others.

It is not only in research that psychiatrists dismiss what their patients tell them, they also do this in clinical practice. Often, they either don't listen or don't ask the appropriate questions about their patients' experience and history and therefore don't find out that the current symptoms are very likely caused by trauma or severe stress, and not by any "psychiatric disorder."

Please note that when I generalise, it does of course not apply to everyone. Some psychiatrists are excellent, but they are in a small minority. It is no wonder that the UK pre-campaign survey found that "the word psychiatrist carried connotations of stigma and even fear."[3] This is understandable, given that psychiatric drugs kill hundreds of thousands of people every year and cripple millions, physically and mentally.[1]

The term "psychiatric survivor" says it all in just two words. In no other medical specialty do the patients call themselves survivors in the sense that they survived *despite* being exposed to that specialty. They fought their way out of a system that is rarely helpful, and which many survivors have described as psychiatric imprisonment, or a facility where there is a door in, but not a door out.

In other medical specialties, the patients are grateful that they survived *because* of the treatments their doctors applied to them. We have never heard of a cardiology survivor or an infectious disease survivor. If you have survived a heart attack, you are not tempted to do the opposite of what your doctor recommends. In psychiatry, you might die if you do what your doctor tells you to do.

Many psychiatric survivors have described how psychiatry, with its excessive use of harmful and ineffective drugs, had stolen 10 or 15 years of their life before they one day decided to take the responsibility for their life back from their psychiatrists and discovered that life is much better without drugs. They often say that what woke them up was that they read some of the books about psychiatry by psychiatrists David Healy, Peter Breggin or Joanna Moncrieff, science journalist Robert Whitaker, or me.

There are thousands of personal stories by psychiatric survivors on the Internet, e.g. on survivingantidepressants.org. In many of them, people explain how they withdrew from psychiatric drugs, one by one, often against their doctor's advice and often with great difficulty, because the drugs had made them dependent and because the psychiatric profession had failed totally in providing proper guidance about how to do it. The psychiatrists have not only been uninterested in tackling this immense problem but have actively denied its existence, as you have just seen and will see much more about in this book.

Mental health issues prevent you from living a full life and they go on in your mind. All patients should be offered psychotherapy, which is also what 75% of them want.[7] However, this is not what they get, which shows once again that the psychiatric profession doesn't listen to its patients. A large US survey of people with depression showed that 87% received depression pills, 23% psychotherapy, 14% anxiety pills, 7% psychosis pills and 5% "mood stabilizers" (a euphemism that the psychiatrists never defined, but they usually mean antiepileptic drugs and lithium, whose main effect is to sedate people).[8]

Most people have issues with their mental health now and then, just as they have issues with their physical health. There is nothing abnormal about that.

Throughout this book, I shall give advice based on the scientific evidence that I have good reasons to believe will lead to better outcomes than if my advice is ignored. But please note that whatever you do and whatever the outcome, you cannot hold me responsible. The information I provide is not a replacement for consultations with healthcare professionals but might empower you to engage in meaningful and informed discussions or to decide to handle the issues yourself. I shall start with a little advice and will give the background for it in the rest of the book:

1. WARNING! Psychiatric drugs are addictive. Never stop them abruptly because withdrawal reactions may consist of severe emotional and physical symptoms that can be dangerous and lead to suicide, violence and homicide.[1]

2. If you have a mental health issue, don't see a psychiatrist. It is too dangerous and might turn out to be the biggest error you made in your entire life.[9]

3. Don't believe what you are told about psychiatric disorders or psychiatric drugs. It is very likely to be wrong.[1]

4. Believe in yourself. You are likely right, and your doctor is wrong. Don't ignore your hunches or feelings. You can easily be led astray if you don't trust yourself.[10]

5. Never let others have responsibility for your life. Stay in control and ask questions. Avoid therapists that are positive toward psychiatric drugs.

6. Your spouse or parent might be your best friend or your worst enemy. They might believe what doctors tell them and might even see it to their advantage to keep you drugged.

Many of the stories I have received from patients have a common theme. The patients had no idea how dangerous it is to become a psychiatric patient and trusted their doctors, willingly following their advice, until they found out years later that their lives had been ruined.

What is particularly diabolic is that the psychological and physical deterioration often occurs gradually, and therefore passes unnoticed, like if you become nearsighted, which you don't discover until one day a friend wonders why you cannot read a road sign close to you. The patients may even be grateful for the drugs they received, although it may be obvious to others that they have been harmed.

Gradual and unnoticed deterioration is not the only problem. A brain under chemical influence may not be able to assess itself. When the brain is numbed by psychoactive substances, the patients may be unaware that they can no longer think clearly or evaluate themselves. This lack of insight into feelings, thoughts and behaviors is called medication spellbinding.[11,12] Medication spellbinding is usually ignored, both by patients and their doctors, which is surprising because we all know that people who have drunk too much cannot judge their ability to drive.

Here is a patient story that illustrates many of the common issues.

A Patient's Psychiatric "Career"

In November 2019, I received an outstanding account from Stine Toft, a Danish patient I met when I lectured for "Better Psychiatry," an organization of relatives to psychiatric patients.[13] Stine was seriously harmed by psychiatric drugs; her life became endangered; and she suffered an excruciating withdrawal phase because she did not receive the necessary guidance. But she is doing well today, aged 44.

Stine gave birth to her second daughter in 2002 after a hard time with "all kinds of trials and hormone treatments." In the aftermath, she wasn't well. She was afraid of losing her daughter and of not being able to protect her well enough. Her doctor diagnosed her with depression, and she was told it was perfectly normal and that she should just take Effexor (venlafaxine, a depression pill) so that her brain would work again—possibly for the rest of her life, but at least for five years.

Her life changed markedly. She put on 110 lbs. (50 kg) and had several weird episodes that she didn't understand. Once she wanted to dig a sandbox for her children, but she ended up putting an entire trampoline two feet into the ground by removing nine cubic yards (seven cubic meters) of soil with a shovel. She also knocked down a wall in the kitchen without warning and without being a craftsman in any way because she felt the family needed a smart conversation kitchen. One day during a job clarification process, she told the job consultant that she wanted to become a lawyer even though she is dyslexic and would never have been able to achieve this.

Stine saw a psychiatrist again, and 15 minutes later the case was clear—she had become bipolar. She was sent for psychoeducation and was told that her condition would definitely last for the rest of her life. She was trained in how to notice even the little things that confirmed that she was ill, and special care was taken to ensure that she took her medicines.

"They managed to put a massive fear in me," Stine wrote, and she clearly identified herself with a sick person who had to tackle life in a certain way in order to survive.

Time passed and she ended up leaving her husband of 15 years. In 2013, she met her current husband, and he asked quite quickly "what the sickness was all about," because he couldn't see it. After a year and a half, she surrendered and agreed to make a small trial with a small withdrawal of the medication. He was happy for that because he had seen several times how disastrous it went when she forgot to take the medication. She once ruined a trip to a summer amusement park because she had forgotten to bring the medicines with her. As the day went on, she got worse and worse with headaches and vomiting; she was confused and just wanted to lie down and sleep until she got the drugs again.

Her medication list included Effexor, later switched to Cymbalta (duloxetine), Lamictal (lamotrigine) and Lyrica (pregabalin), two anti-epileptics, and Seroquel (quetiapine, a psychosis pill). In addition, she was given medication for the adverse effects caused by the drugs and for her metabolic problem.

This is a dangerous cocktail. Depression pills double the risk of suicide, not only in children but also in adults,[1,14-18] antiepileptics also double the risk of suicide,[19] and both depression pills and antiepileptics can make people manic,[18,19] which happened to her and resulted in an erroneous diagnosis of having become bipolar.

The withdrawal process took two and a half years, with her husband helping the best he could to make the process as gentle as possible. They did not understand it at the time, but discovered along the way, what the receptor saturation curve means, namely that you need to reduce the dose by less and less the further you come down. Extremely few doctors are aware of this,[20] and most official recommendations are outright dangerous, e.g. they may say that you should reduce the dose by 50% every two weeks when you taper depression pills.[21] Thus, already after two reductions, you are down to only 25% of the starting dose, which is far too quickly for most patients.

Stine's life became endangered. She was scared to death that it would end badly and was often thinking about giving up. She introduced several pauses in the process. Thoughts of suicide were extremely pressing during the times when she tapered, because it was absolutely horrible.

Inexplicably, Stine had accepted that she obviously hated life and wanted to put an end to it. She is otherwise an energetic person who loves life and had never had suicidal thoughts until she started taking drugs, nor after stopping them. But the withdrawal process was completely "crazy," and she often considered whether taking her own life would be more humane.

During withdrawal, she had some "wildly weird experiences." On the good end, she took it upon herself several times just to listen to nature and the birds. It was a powerful experience, because she could not remember when she had last experienced this in the years she was "doped." A little sadder were the other symptoms that came during withdrawal. The abstinence symptoms included dives that could easily be interpreted as depression, and during withdrawal of Lyrica, she was anxious and felt life was unbearable. One morning in the bath she began to cry, because just feeling the water on her body was something she had not noted for many years.

At this point in time, she became aware of two of my books about psychiatry[1,22] and realized that everything she had experienced was well known and perfectly normal. It was really shocking to her to read about how it is normal practice to be exposed to the hell she had been through, but also liberating to discover that it is normal; that she probably wasn't sick; and that there was nothing wrong with her.

By the end of the withdrawal, she had a strange experience where, for about half a year, she was almost crooked in her body. She constantly had a feeling of tipping to the left and had a hard time walking straight. During several periods, other muscle groups failed. When she once played a game where a stick is thrown after wooden blocks, her hand didn't release the stick.

After withdrawal, things started to get better, and she wanted to work again, even though she had been out of the job market for many years and was on disability pension. She planned to take a business driver's license and drive a taxi, but "Oh no, oh no! There was a big no from the police." They sent a letter stating that her driver's license was time limited and that she would need to provide documentation every two years that she wasn't sick.

"The fact that they chose to throw an extra diagnosis after someone who is on depression pills is pretty terrible," she wrote. "Today, I must renew my driver's license every two years for that reason. But you wouldn't imagine how hard it was to avoid that they took it away completely. When I contacted psychiatry because of my contact with the police, they first refused to see me—because I was well. So, I couldn't get their help to prove I wasn't sick and thus fit to drive. After intense pressure from me, my own doctor finally persuaded them to take me in for a talk and make a statement, which dryly noted that my 'illness' wasn't active. I could have strangled them, because that means I'm still sick and, in the eyes of the police, one that needs to be monitored in future."

Stine completely disagrees with the bipolar diagnosis. She never had manic episodes before starting on the medication, and never had them after she quit. But the diagnosis is glued to her for the rest of her life, although it is well known that depression pills can trigger mania and thus cause the psychiatrists to make a wrong diagnosis, confusing the drug harm with a new illness.

> It is medical malpractice to make a new diagnosis, as if
> there is something wrong with the patient, when the
> condition could be a harm caused by the medication.
> Psychiatrists do this all the time.

Stine gave up the idea of becoming a taxi driver. She became a
coach and went on studying to become a psychotherapist. She works
with many different people and helps patients taper off their depression
pills, with great success. They are reclaiming life and seeing it move
forward. She knows it is important to support them when they
withdraw so that they will not face the same troubles as she did. There
are many thoughts and fears, and many people have difficulty defining
themselves if they are no longer sick. The combination of tapering and
therapy seems to have an extremely beneficial effect.

It is difficult to convince people that stopping their drugs is a good
idea. Many passionately believe in them, because they have been told
they are sick, and there is often great pressure from their relatives. Stine
experienced herself what it means to stand alone with the withdrawal.
Today, she no longer sees her family. They maintained the claim that
she was ill and just needed to take her medication. This mistaken view
is nourished by the fact that three-quarters of websites even today still
falsely claim that people fall ill with depression because of a chemical
imbalance in their brain (see below).[23] If you believe in this bogus, you
also believe that you cannot do without the medicine.

A few years ago, Stine bought the domain name medicin-fri.dk
(medicine-free.dk) because she wants to provide information about
taking drugs and their harms, in cooperation with others, as well as
provide help and support for withdrawal.

Too few people know about the problems or have ever heard of
them. Stine wants to change that and wants to make sure that she does
not give incorrect advice and information. She therefore wrote to me
and asked if I knew others who would like to join an organized
network about these issues.

In addition to her daily work with clients, Stine lectures, but finds it
difficult to "be allowed" to get the message out. She has lectured for
Psychiatry in the Capital Region about being bipolar, which was easy,
as everyone wants to see a sick person and hear her story. But a success
story that calls the system into question is not interesting.

Stine is passionate about changing things and has, for example,
established several self-help groups; lectured for the Depression

Association; volunteered in the Red Cross; started groups for lonely people; and mentored young people.

She suggested to Better Psychiatry in her hometown that they invite me to lecture. They didn't know who I was, and the chairwoman introduced the meeting by saying that if more money was allotted to psychiatry it would probably be okay. I started my lecture by saying I wasn't sure this was a good idea. If more money came in, even more diagnoses would be made, even more drugs would be used, and even more people would end up on disability pension because they cannot function when they are drugged.[24]

Stine wants to lecture on the theme, "Surviving Psychiatry." She finds it overwhelming to live a life that, after so many years on medication, she thought was completely out of reach. Although her past life was "foolishly handled by various psychiatrists and other well-meaning doctors," she doesn't want to mess it up by asking for access to her files. She would rather look ahead and inform others via websites and lectures about how harmful it is to blindly become medicated—often for no reason at all.

Stine is convinced that virtually none of her strange experiences during the 14 years she was drugged would have happened if she had not been given medication. Her memory suffered a severe blow, but it is improving.

She cannot understand why her doctors didn't stop the drugging. Nothing could justify her massive drugging, and even when she gained weight from 155 to 265 lbs. (70 to 120 kg), the doctors didn't respond, besides giving her medication to increase the metabolism, which was "completely nuts... extremely disabling in every conceivable way and in itself almost something they could give a depression diagnosis for, because it was a sad thing to expose your body to."

Stine considers the system to be hopeless. The colossal overuse of psychoactive drugs produces chronic patients, often based on temporary problems,[24] as I shall explain in the following.

2 Is Psychiatry Evidence-Based?

Psychiatry was in a state of crisis in the United States in the middle of the last century because psychologists were more popular than psychiatrists.[1] The psychiatric guild therefore decided to make psychiatry a medical specialty, which would make psychiatrists look like real doctors and delineate them from psychologists who were not allowed to prescribe drugs.

Ever since, massive propaganda, fraud, manipulations with the research data, hiding suicides and other deaths, and lies in drug marketing have paved the way for the illusion that psychiatry is a respectable discipline that provides drugs that cure patients.[1-4]

As explained in the first chapter, the "customers," the patients and their relatives, do not agree with the salespeople. When this is the case, the providers are usually quick to change their products or services, but this doesn't happen in psychiatry, which has a monopoly on treating patients with mental health issues, with family doctors as their complacent frontline sales staff that do not ask uncomfortable questions about what they are selling.

The family doctor is most people's port of entry into psychiatry. This is where sad, worried, stressed or burned-out people address their symptoms. The doctor rarely allots the necessary time to inquire about the events that caused the patient to end up in this situation. The consultation often ends after a few minutes with a diagnosis, which might not be correct, and a prescription for one or more psychiatric drugs, although talk therapy might have been better. A study in the United States showed that over half the physicians wrote prescriptions after discussing depression with patients for three minutes or less.[5]

You might get a psychiatric drug even if there is no good reason to prescribe it for you, e.g. a depression pill for insomnia, problems at school, exam anxiety, harassment at work, marital abuse, break-up with a boyfriend, bereavement, economic problems, or divorce. This is also common if you see a psychiatrist.

In contrast to other medical specialties, psychiatry is built on a number of myths, which have been rejected so firmly by good research that it is appropriate to call them lies. I therefore warn you again. Most of what you have been told or will ever hear about psychiatry, psychiatric drugs, electroshock, and forced admission and treatment, is wrong. This has been documented in numerous research articles and books.[1-11]

Here is some general advice, which will lead to better outcomes than if it is ignored:

1. It is rarely a good idea to see a family doctor if you have a mental health issue. As doctors are trained in using drugs, you will most likely be harmed. If not in the short term, then in the long term.

2. If you get a prescription from your family doctor for a psychiatric drug, don't go to the pharmacy.

3. Find someone who is good at talk therapy, e.g. a psychologist. If you cannot afford it or if there is a long waiting list, then remember it is usually better to do nothing than to see your doctor.

4. Consider if you need a social counsellor or a lawyer. Doctors cannot help you with a broken marriage, for example, and pills won't help you either.

Let's have a closer look at what is wrong with current-day psychiatry. Psychiatrists claim that their specialty is built on the biopsychosocial model of disease that takes biology, psychology, and socio-environmental factors into account when trying to explain why people fall ill.

The reality is vastly different. Biological psychiatry has been the predominant disease model ever since the president of the US Society of Biological Psychiatry, Harold Himwich, in 1955 came up with the totally absurd idea that psychosis pills work like insulin for diabetes.[9]

It even seems to be getting worse. Fifteen years ago, some of psychiatry's spokespersons were more concerned than today's leaders about the dangers of being too close to the drug industry. Steven Sharfstein, president of the American Psychiatric Association, wrote in 2005:

> "As we address these Big Pharma issues, we must examine the fact that as a profession, we have allowed the biopsychosocial model to become the bio-bio-bio model... Drug company representatives bearing gifts are frequent visitors to psychiatrists' offices and consulting rooms. We should have the wisdom and distance to call these gifts what they are—kickbacks and bribes... If we are seen as mere pill pushers and employees of the pharmaceutical industry, our credibility as a profession is compromised."[12]

Other statements were less fortunate: "Pharmaceutical companies have developed and brought to market medications that have transformed the lives of millions of psychiatric patients." Sure, but not for the better.

"The proven effectiveness of antidepressant, mood-stabilizing, and antipsychotic medications has helped sensitize the public to the reality of mental illness and taught them that treatment works. In this way, Big Pharma has helped reduce stigma associated with psychiatric treatment and with psychiatrists."

The treatments do not provide worthwhile effects, particularly not when their harms are considered as well, and the stigma has increased.[4] But that's how the psychiatric leaders fool people. A systematic review of 33 studies found that biogenetic causal attributions weren't associated with more tolerant attitudes; they were related to stronger rejection in most studies examining schizophrenia.[13] Biological pseudo-explanations increase perceived dangerousness, fear and desire for distance from patients with schizophrenia because they make people believe that the patients are unpredictable,[13-16] and they also lead to reductions in clinicians' empathy and to social exclusion.[17]

The biological model generates undue pessimism about the chances of recovery and reduces efforts to change, compared to a psychosocial explanation. Many patients describe discrimination as more long-lasting and disabling than the psychosis itself, and a major barrier to recovery.[14,15] Patients and their families experience more stigma and discrimination from mental health professionals than from any other sector of society, and over 80% of people with the schizophrenia label think that the diagnosis itself is damaging and dangerous. Therefore, some psychiatrists now avoid using the term schizophrenia.[15]

Sharfstein admitted that, "there is less psychotherapy provided by psychiatrists than 10 years ago. This is true despite the strong evidence base that many psychotherapies are effective used alone or in combination with medications." What a tragedy this is. This is not the progress we hear so much about.

Sharfstein couldn't resist the temptation of playing the "antipsychiatry" card: "responding to the antipsychiatry remarks… one of the charges against psychiatry… is that many patients are being prescribed the wrong drugs or drugs they don't need. These charges are true, but it is not psychiatry's fault—it is the fault of the broken health care system that the United States appears to be willing to endure."

Of course. All the harms psychiatrists cause by overdosing entire populations are NEVER their fault, but someone else's.

Psychiatrist Niall McLaren has written a very instructive book with many patient stories telling us that anxiety is a key symptom in psychiatry.[11] If a psychiatrist or family doctor doesn't take a very careful history, they might miss that the current episode of distress, which they diagnose as depression, started as anxiety many years earlier when the patient was a teenager. They should therefore have dealt with the anxiety with talk therapy instead of handing out pills.

Niall has developed a standard way with which he approaches all new patients in order not to overlook anything important. It takes time, but the time invested initially pays back many times over and leads to better outcomes for his patients than the standard approach in psychiatry.

Niall has an interest in philosophy but has been met with extreme hostility when he challenged his colleagues by asking them what the foundation was for their biological model of psychiatric disorders. There is none. In his own words:[11]

"So we can forget biological psychiatry. Trouble is, an awful lot of people have an awful lot of money invested in giving biological treatments for mental disorder, and they won't give it up without a fight. Worse still, there's an awful lot of high-flying academic psychiatrists around the world who have invested their entire careers, and their egos (which is much worse), in claiming that mental disorder is biological in nature. They will fight tenaciously to save their jobs and their reputations. So we're stuck with biological psychiatry for a while. Just because it has been proven wrong doesn't mean it will fade away overnight. The value of biological psychiatry is that it isn't necessary to talk to a patient beyond asking a few standard questions to work out which disease he has, and that can easily be done by a nurse armed with a questionnaire. This will give a diagnosis which then dictates the drugs he should have."

Biological psychiatry assumes that specific diagnoses exist that result from specific changes in the brain, and that there are specific drugs that correct these changes, which are therefore beneficial. We shall look at these assumptions one by one.

Are Psychiatric Diagnoses Specific and Reliable?

Psychiatric diagnoses are neither specific, nor reliable.[4,6,18,19] They are highly unspecific, and psychiatrists disagree wildly when asked to diagnose the same patients independently of each other. There are few such studies, and their results were so embarrassing for the American Psychiatric Association that they buried them so deeply that it required extensive detective work to find them.[19] The funeral took place in a smoke of positive rhetoric in surprisingly short articles, given the importance of the subject. Even the largest study, of 592 people, was disappointing although the investigators took great care in training the assessors.[20]

Psychiatric diagnoses are not built on science but are consensus-type exercises where it is decided by a show of hands which symptoms should be included in a diagnostic test.[18] This checklist approach is like the familiar parlor game, Find Five Errors. A person who has at least five symptoms out of nine is declared depressed.

If we look hard enough, we will find "errors" in all people. There is nothing objective and verifiable about this way of making diagnoses, which are derived from an arbitrary constellation of symptoms. How many criteria and which ones do we vote for need to be present to make a given diagnosis?

I lecture a lot for various audiences, both professionals and lay people, and I often expose people to the recommended test for adult ADHD (attention deficit hyperactivity disorder).[4,21] It never fails. Between one-third and one-half of the audience test positive. When I tested my wife, she scored a full house, which is six out of six criteria. Only four positive replies to the questionnaire are needed for the diagnosis. Once, when one of my daughters and her boyfriend visited us for dinner, we discussed the silliness of psychiatric diagnoses and to illustrate it, I subjected them to the test. My daughter scored five, like I did, and her very laid-back boyfriend whom I would never suspect would be positive, scored four. So, we were four people enjoying our dinner and company, all with a bogus psychiatric diagnosis.

My little exercise makes people realize how foolish and unscientific psychiatric diagnoses are. I always tell people that I am in the same boat as them and that they shouldn't worry but be happy, as the song by Bobby McFerrin goes, because some of the most interesting people I have ever met qualify for the ADHD diagnosis. They are dynamic and creative and have difficulty sitting still on their chairs pretending they are listening if the lecturer is dull. Yet, the psychiatrists have had the barefaced impudence to tell the whole world that people with an ADHD diagnosis suffer from a "neurodevelopmental disorder," e.g. the Diagnostic and Statistical Manual of Mental Disorders (DSM-5) used in USA, and the International Classification of Diseases (ICD-11) used in Europe both say this.

> To postulate that billions of people have wrong brains is as outrageous as it gets.

One of the times I lectured for "Better psychiatry," a woman in the audience said: "I have ADHD." I replied: "No, you haven't. You can have a dog, a car, or a boyfriend, but you cannot have ADHD. It is a social construct." I explained it is just a label, not something that exists in nature, like an elephant everyone can see. People tend to think they get an explanation for their troubles when psychiatrists give them a name, but this is circular reasoning. Paul behaves in a certain way, and we will give this behavior a name, ADHD. Poul behaves this way because he has ADHD. Logically, it is impossible to argue this way.

I often joked during my lectures that we also need a diagnosis for those children who are *too* good at sitting still and not make themselves seen or heard in class. This became true, with the invention of the diagnosis ADD, attention deficit disorder, without the hyperactivity. From that day on, I have joked about how long we shall wait before we will also see a diagnosis for those in the middle, because then there will be a drug for everyone and the drug industry will have reached their ultimate goal, that no one will escape being treated.

The depression diagnosis isn't much better. It is very easy to get this diagnosis even though you are not really depressed but just feel a little beside your usual self.[4]

Even the more serious diagnoses are highly uncertain. Many people—in some studies by far most of them – have been considered on revision to have been wrongly diagnosed with schizophrenia.[4]

Given this immense uncertainty, disagreement, and arbitrariness, it should be very easy to get rid of a wrong diagnosis. However, it's impossible, and there is no court of appeal like in criminal cases. It is like in medieval times where people were condemned for no reason and with no possibility of appeal. As you will see in the section about forced treatment in Chapter 4, the law is routinely being violated, which we would not tolerate in any other sector of society.

It doesn't seem to matter whether a diagnosis is correct or wrong. It follows you for the rest of your life and can make it difficult to get the education you dream about, a job, certain pensions, to become approved for adoption or even just to keep your driver's licence.[22,23] Furthermore, psychiatric diagnoses are frequently being abused in child custody cases when the parents get divorced.[22] Even when the diagnosis is obviously wrong and the psychiatrist herself seriously doubted it when she made it, you cannot have it removed.[23] It sticks to you forever, like if you were a branded cow.

Danish filmmaker Anahi Testa Pedersen made the film, "Diagnosing Psychiatry,"[24] about my attempts at creating a better psychiatry and about her own struggles with the system. She got the diagnosis schizotypy, which is a very vague and highly dubious concept (see Chapter 5), when she was admitted to a psychiatric ward due to severe distress over a divorce. It was obvious that she suffered from acute distress and should never have had a psychiatric diagnosis or been treated with drugs, but at the ward they gave her Seroquel, a psychosis pill, and Lexapro, a depression pill. Anahi was deeply shocked to learn that even though she had voluntarily contacted the psychiatric ward, the doors were locked behind her. When she questioned her diagnosis at discharge, she was told: "Here, we make diagnoses!"[22] The drugs doped her and made her indifferent, and she withdrew from them.

Another shock came eight years later when she received a letter from Psychiatry in the Capital Region. They wanted to examine her daughter. They believed that psychiatric disorders are inherited and that it is therefore likely that children of the mentally ill will also become ill.

Anahi became angry. Her daughter is well functioning, happy, healthy and has many friends. The summons came without her being asked about her course after discharge, or her daughter's situation and well-being, and the letter stigmatized both her and her daughter. She phoned a psychiatrist at the department where she had stayed eight years previously, but even though her family doctor assured her that she was well and that it was remarkable that she got the diagnosis in the first place, she was also told, by the psychiatrist, when she asked for a re-examination: "The system doesn't do that!" She was left with a lifetime, yet erroneous, sentence. This wouldn't have happened if she had been wrongly sentenced for a crime, but in psychiatry, this is perfectly "normal."

> The sticking diagnosis problem is an awfully good reason not to see a psychiatrist. YOU MUST AVOID GETTING A DIAGNOSIS.

Psychiatry's Starter Kit: Depression Pills

Patients and their relatives commonly refer to depression pills as "Psychiatry's Starter Kit." This is because many people start their psychiatric "careers" by consulting their family doctor with some problem many of us have from time to time and leave the doctor's office with a prescription for a depression pill, which brings them into trouble.

As already noted, depression pills are often prescribed for non-approved indications, so-called *off-label* use. When the problems accumulate, the family doctor may refer the patient to psychiatric treatment. Most of these problems are iatrogenic (Greek for caused by a doctor). If you read package inserts for depression pills, which are easy to find in a Google search, e.g. *duloxetine fda*, you will see that these drugs make some people hypomanic, manic, or psychotic in other ways. When this happens, your doctor will likely conclude that you have become bipolar or suffer from psychotic depression and will give you additional drugs, e.g. a psychosis pill, lithium, an antiepileptic drug, or all three, in addition to the depression pill.

There is considerable overlap between the harms of psychiatric drugs and the symptoms psychiatrists use when making diagnoses, so it may not take long before you have several diagnoses and are on several drugs. [2,4]

In 2015, I was invited to lecture at a major hospital in Denmark by the psychiatric organisation in that region. Rasmus Licht, professor of psychiatry, lectured after me and there was a general discussion.

Rasmus is a specialist in bipolar disorder, and I was one of the examiners when he defended his PhD about mania 17 years earlier.

I asked him how he could know, when he made the diagnosis bipolar in a patient who received a drug for ADHD, that it was not just the drug harms he saw because they are very similar to the symptoms doctors use when diagnosing bipolar. I was flabbergasted when he said that a psychiatrist was able to distinguish between these two possibilities. I decided not to go any further into the discussion.

Rasmus said a lot else that wasn't correct, which illustrated what psychiatry does to its own people. When I first met him, he was a bright young man who impressed me. I hadn't seen him in all those years, and it was shocking to watch how he had assimilated all psychiatry's wrong ideas. We corresponded a little afterwards in a very friendly manner, but my attempts at convincing him he was wrong failed.

One of the things Rasmus wrote was that, "no matter what you write, it has not been clearly shown that antidepressants can change [sic] bipolar disorder. This has been believed, which is why it is mentioned in ICD-10 and DSM-IV that if the mania only occurs when the patient has received an antidepressant at the same time, it speaks against bipolar disorder, as it is understood it could be drug induced mania. However, in contrast, the DSM-5 has taken the consequences of recent epidemiological studies and written that, even though a mania occurs during treatment with an antidepressant, this should be perceived as a true, i.e. primary, bipolar disorder. So, in this case, you speak against better knowledge."

I wondered how it was possible for Rasmus to believe in such nonsense. It is total baloney to postulate that a mania that occurs during treatment with a depression pill is a new disorder when it might as well be a iatrogenic harm. It is nothing else than a smart trick psychiatrists use to distance themselves from the harms they cause and from their accountability. It is always the patient who is to blame, never us or our drugs, is the message they send.

Rasmus should have criticized the psychiatrists who made up the DSM-5 in such a way that they were beyond reproach. Think also of Stine Toft whose history I described in the first chapter. She has never been manic, apart from the time when she received a depression pill.

I have had many such experiences, which is why I see absolutely no hope for psychiatry. People with mental health issues should consult professionals who will not treat them with psychiatric drugs but will listen to them and help them in other ways.[25]

I have described elsewhere how devastating the psychiatrists' self-inflicted blindness towards reality is for their patients.[4] The most prominent American child psychiatrist, Joseph Biederman, is also one of the most harmful ones. He invented the diagnosis juvenile bipolar disorder, and he and his co-workers made a diagnosis of bipolar in 23% of 128 children with ADHD.[26] This condition was virtually unknown before Biederman stepped into the scene, but in just eight years, from 1994-95 to 2002-03, the number of medical visits in the United States for children diagnosed with bipolar disorder increased 40-fold (an increase of 3900%).[27]

Do Patients Fall Ill Because of a Chemical Imbalance in the Brain?

There are no specific chemical changes in the brain that cause psychiatric disorders. The studies that have claimed that a common mental disorder like depression and psychosis starts with a chemical imbalance in the brain are all unreliable.[4]

A difference in dopamine levels between patients with a schizophrenia diagnosis and healthy people cannot tell us anything about what started the psychosis. If a house burns down and we find ashes, it doesn't mean that it was the ashes that set the house on fire. Similarly, if a lion attacks us, we get terribly frightened and produce stress hormones, but this doesn't prove that it was the stress hormones that made us scared. People with psychoses have often suffered traumatic experiences in the past, so we should see these trauma as contributing causal factors and not reduce suffering to some biochemical imbalance that, if it exists at all, is more likely to be the result of the psychosis rather than its cause.[28]

A paper that analyzed the 41 most rigorous studies found that people who had suffered childhood adversity were 2.8 times more likely to develop psychosis than those who had not ($p < 0.001$, which means that the probability of getting such a result, or an even larger number than 2.8, if in reality there is no relationship, is less than one in a thousand).[29] Nine of the ten studies that tested for a dose-response relationship found it.[29] Another study found that people who had experienced three types of trauma (e.g. sexual abuse, physical abuse and bullying) were 18 times more likely to be psychotic than non-abused people, and if they had experienced five types of trauma, they were 193 times more likely to be psychotic (95% 51 to 736 times, which means that the true risk is 95% likely to be within the interval 51 to 736 times the risk of a person who has not been exposed to trauma).[30]

Such data are very convincing unless you are a psychiatrist. A survey of 2813 UK psychiatrists showed that for every psychiatrist who thinks schizophrenia is caused primarily by social factors there are 115 who think it is caused primarily by biological factors.[31]

The myth about a chemical imbalance in the brain being the cause of psychiatric disorders is one of the biggest lies in psychiatry and also one of the most harmful ones. As noted above, it has existed for at least 65 years, since Himwich claimed that psychosis pills work like insulin for diabetes.[9] It seems impossible to make the myth go away, as it is so useful for the psychiatric guild to keep it. It gives them an alibi for treating their patients with harmful drugs and makes them look like real doctors in the public eye.

In 2019, Maryanne Demasi and I collected information about depression from 39 popular websites in 10 countries: Australia, Canada, Denmark, Ireland, New Zealand, Norway, South Africa, Sweden, UK, and USA. We found that 29 websites (74%) attributed depression to a chemical imbalance or claimed that depression pills could fix or correct such an imbalance.[32]

I have good reasons for calling my 2015 psychiatry book, *Deadly Psychiatry and Organised Denial*.[4] The denial, not only of reality but even of psychiatry's own stance when challenged, is so immense that I shall illustrate it in some detail, using my own country as an example. It is the same everywhere, so it doesn't matter if you have never heard of the people I mention.

In 2005, psychiatry professor Lars Kessing and colleagues published a survey of 493 patients with depressive or bipolar disorder that showed that 80% of the patients agreed with the statement: "Antidepressants correct the changes that occurred in my brain due to stress or problems."[33] I shall say more about Kessing in Chapter 5 where I shall also describe what happens when critical TV programs try to tell the truth about psychiatry.[34-36]

In 2013, Thomas Middelboe, the chairman of the Danish Psychiatric Association, described the term chemical imbalance as a metaphor psychiatry has grasped in an attempt to explain diseases whose causes are unknown:[37] "It is a bit goofy to say that people lack a substance in the brain, but chemical imbalance—I might use that term. We are dealing with neurobiological processes that are disturbed."

In 2014, I debated with psychiatry professor Poul Videbech at a public meeting arranged by medical students. After I had carefully explained and documented why far too many people are in treatment with depression pills and had suggested that we taper off the drugs, Videbech said, in front of 600 people including patients and their relatives: "Who would take insulin from a diabetic?"

In 2015, Psychiatry in the Capital Region and the Joint Council of Psychiatric Societies held a meeting with the title, "Truths or falsehoods about psychiatric drugs." The occasion was that I had started a prolonged debate about psychiatric drugs a year earlier when I published ten myths in psychiatry that are harmful for the patients in a newspaper.[4] The article also exists in English.[38] Officially, the aim of the meeting was to provide "a neutral and sober assessment of the drugs," but its true purpose was to protect the status quo. There was a long introduction where my name wasn't mentioned even though I was the direct reason for having the meeting, and I wasn't invited to speak. Psychologist Olga Runciman pointed out that the story about mental disorders being caused by a chemical imbalance was dead abroad and asked if it was also dead in Denmark. None of the psychiatry professors wanted to answer, and the chair didn't hold them to account, not even after I had said twice that they hadn't replied.

Eight months later, the day before my psychiatry book came out,[4] there was a long interview with me in the newspaper where I had described the ten myths.[39] I emphasized that one of the biggest myths, which over half of patients had been told,[33] is that they suffer from a chemical imbalance in the brain. I also said that many patients ended up taking drugs for the rest of their lives because they had been fooled this way or had been told that they would become brain damaged if they didn't take the drugs.

Videbech was also interviewed and said: "Against better knowledge, he assigns to his opponent all sorts of unfair motives. For example, we have known for the last 20 years that the theory of the chemical imbalance in the brain for depression is far too simple. I have written about this in my textbooks for many years. It is therefore totally off limits when I and others are assigned such views."

Well, not really. The myth about the chemical imbalance is only a thing of the past when challenged. Psychiatry professor Birte Glenthøj was also interviewed and confirmed that the myth was still alive and well: "We know from research that patients suffering from schizophrenia have on average increased formation and release of dopamine, and that this is linked to the development of the psychotic symptoms. Increased dopamine activity is also seen before patients are first given antipsychotic medication, so it has nothing to do with the medication."

Two weeks after I published my psychiatry book, psychiatrist Marianne Geoffroy wrote in an industry supported throwaway magazine that I used public funds to publish private, non-scientific books, which she compared to Scientology books. She claimed that I scared citizens suffering from psychiatric disorders away from getting relevant treatment.[40] In an electronic comment, psychiatrist Lars Søndergård (see more about him in Chapter 5) said that he didn't know of any psychiatrist who attributed mental illness to a "chemical imbalance in the brain".

Another psychiatrist, Julius Nissen, responded: "I have spent my many years in psychiatry talking to a lot of people who have received exactly this explanation and the comparison with insulin, that it is a substance they need. This conviction makes it very hard to motivate them to withdraw from the drug. It is precisely because they, during the withdrawal, de facto experience a 'chemical imbalance,' now that the brain is accustomed to the substance. They therefore feel confirmed that the hypothesis is true because they are ill, even though it is side effects that must be overcome."

In early 2017, Videbech postulated again that when people are depressed, there is an imbalance in the brain.[41] I complained to the editor of the publicly available *Handbook for Patients*, which has official status in Denmark, that Kessing and Videbech had written in their two contributions that depression is caused by a chemical imbalance.[42,43]

I got nowhere, of course, but felt it was my duty towards the patients to at least try. Kessing and Videbech changed a few minor things and introduced new claims that made their articles worse. I complained again, and again to no avail, and the lie about the chemical imbalance continued.

In his update, Kessing added that, "it is known that antidepressant drugs stimulate the brain to make new nerve cells in certain areas." Videbech wrote the same, but there were no references. If this can happen, it only means that depression pills are harmful to brain cells, as the brain forms new cells in response to a brain injury. This is well documented, for example for electroshock therapy and psychosis pills.[7]

Leading psychiatrists consider their patients ignorant, but I must say that the level of ignorance among themselves about their own specialty is astounding.

Like Kessing, Videbech argued that treatment with depression pills can be lifelong, e.g. if the depression appears after 50 years of age. I have never heard of any reliable scientific evidence in support of this.

In 2018, a patient wrote in a newspaper:[44] "When a psychiatrist changed my medication... it 'worked' by putting on about 20 kilos (44 lbs.). When I wanted to come off the drug, he told me the usual lie: That I had a chemical imbalance and needed the pills. So, I continued... My mother always said, 'don't go to the bakery for meat.' And going to a medically trained doctor in the hope of getting answers to mental problems is exactly that." Subsequently, my PhD student Anders Sørensen helped him come off his drugs.

Why is it that we need to listen to the patients and not to the psychiatrists if we want to know the truth about psychiatric drugs and electroshock?[4,23] One patient couldn't remember even the commonest things, like the name of the Danish capital, after she was electroshocked.[23] She was permanently and seriously brain damaged by electroshocks she should never have received but she was told it was her "disease" even though she didn't have any psychiatric disorder; she was sexually abused as a child. Her book is a frightening account of virtually everything that is wrong with psychiatry,[23] just as the book about a young woman the psychiatrists killed with psychosis pills (see Chapter 4).[4,45]

Before turning to the question whether psychiatric drugs have specific, worthwhile effects, in line with the doctrine of biological psychiatry, I shall expose the idea about a chemical imbalance to a little logic.

If a deficit in serotonin is the cause of depression and a drug that increases serotonin works for depression, then we would not expect a drug that lowers serotonin to work. Nonetheless, this is the case, e.g. for tianeptine.[2,3] More generally, it seems that almost everything that causes side effects, which all drugs do, "works" for depression,[8] including several drugs that do not increase serotonin, e.g. Remeron (mirtazapine). This, and other evidence I shall discuss below, suggests that depression pills don't work for depression. The patients think they are helpful because they can feel something is happening in their body, and the psychiatrists delude themselves.

If a deficit in serotonin is the cause of depression, mice genetically depleted of brain serotonin should be seriously depressed, but they behave just like other mice.[46]

If a deficit in serotonin is the cause of depression, depression pills should work pretty quickly because monoamine levels in the brain increase in one to two days after the start of treatment.[47] They don't. The improvement comes gradually, with very little difference between drug and placebo, and whether they get drug or placebo, it usually takes weeks before the patients can feel their depression has lifted.[4,48]

If depression pills work by increasing the level of serotonin, we would not expect them to work in diseases that have never been claimed to have anything to do with a lack of serotonin, e.g. social phobia.[47] When my research group reviewed the type of diagnoses that had been investigated in placebo-controlled trials of depression pills, we counted 214 unique diagnoses, in addition to depression and anxiety.[49] The trials were driven by commercial interests, focusing on prevalent diseases and everyday problems to such an extent that no one can live a full life without experiencing several of the problems for which these drugs were tested. We concluded that depression pills are the modern version of Aldous Huxley's soma pill intended to keep everyone happy in *Brave New World*.

In 1996, Steven Hyman, former director of the US National Institute of Mental Health, pointed out that depression pills do not correct a chemical imbalance in the brain but, on the contrary, create a chemical imbalance.[50] This is why so many people struggle to come off psychiatric drugs (see Chapter 4). The myth about the chemical imbalance is very harmful for other reasons. It makes people believe there is something seriously wrong with them, and sometimes they are even told it is hereditary. The result is that patients fear what would happen if they stopped, even if they taper off slowly. Similarly, the myth convinces doctors they are right when they persuade their patients to take drugs they don't like or are afraid of.

The drug industry and its paid allies in the psychiatric profession have betrayed the whole world, and the recipe is simple. You take a drug and find out that it increases X, e.g. serotonin, or lowers Y, e.g. dopamine. You then invent the hypothesis that the people you treat are deficient in X or produce too much Y. There is nothing wrong with inventing hypotheses. That's how science works. But when your hypothesis gets rejected, again and again, no matter what you do and how ingenious you are and how much you manipulate your design and the data, it is time to bury the hypothesis for good.

This won't happen. The chemical imbalance myth is not a question about science, it is about money, prestige, and guild interests.

Can you imagine a cardiologist saying, "You have a chemical imbalance in your heart, so you need to take this drug for the rest of your life," when she doesn't have a clue what she is talking about?

Are Psychoactive Drugs Specific and Worthwhile?

The psychiatrists constantly say that they use drugs with specific effects that are similarly effective as many other drugs, e.g. used for rheumatic pain and asthma.

For many psychiatric drugs, we can tell which main receptor in the brain they target, resulting in blocking or enhancing the effect of a particular neurotransmitter, e.g. serotonin, dopamine or gammaamino-butyric acid (GABA).

This looks like a specific effect, like insulin for diabetes, but it isn't. If your blood sugar is very high, you may end up in hyperglycemic coma, which can lead to permanent brain damage and death. However, if you are treated with insulin, intravenous fluids, and electrolytes, you will usually recover fully. The effect is dramatic and quick.

Antibiotics are also highly specific treatments. You may become fatally ill if you are infected with streptococci but may recover within an hour or two if you receive penicillin.

Psychiatric drugs interact with several receptors and there are receptors elsewhere in the body, outside the brain. More than a hundred neuro-transmitters have been described, and the brain is a highly complicated system, which makes it impossible to know what will happen when you perturb this system with a drug.

It is revealing to see what happens when people are exposed to psychiatric drugs and other brain-active substances. There are remarkable similarities, no matter which drug or substance we use, whether it be prescription drugs, narcotics bought in the street, alcohol or opium. Common effects are numbing of feelings, emotional blunting, drowsiness, lack of control over your thoughts, caring less about yourself and others, and reduced or absent capacity for having sex and falling in love.

Psychoactive substances change your brain and if you abruptly stop taking a drug, the withdrawal symptoms are also remarkably similar, no matter what drug it is. There are also differences, but it is clear that psychiatric drugs do not have specific actions. If you give them to healthy volunteers or animals, they will experience the same unspecific effects as patients do. This is not so for specific drugs. If you give penicillin to a healthy person, that person will not become any better and will likely not feel anything.

We have many specific drugs that can increase survival. Antibiotics, antihypertensives, streptokinase for heart attacks, aspirin for preventing new heart attacks, coagulation factors for people with hereditary clotting defects, vitamins for people with serious vitamin deficiencies, thyroid hormones for myxedema, and a lot else.

Psychiatric drugs cannot cure people, only dampen their symptoms, which come with a lot of harmful effects. And they don't save people's lives; they kill people. I have estimated, based on the best science I could find, that psychiatric drugs are the third leading cause of death, after heart disease and cancer.[4] Perhaps they are not quite that harmful, but there is no doubt that they kill hundreds of thousands of people every year. I have estimated that just one psychosis pill, Zyprexa (olanzapine), had killed 200,000 patients up to 2007.[51] What is particularly saddening is that by far most of these patients should never have been treated with Zyprexa.

Do the psychiatrists want to hear about this? No. In October 2017, I gave two invited talks at the World Psychiatric Association's 17th World Congress of Psychiatry in Berlin. When I spoke about "Withdrawal from psychotropics," there were around 150 psychiatrists in the audience. Fifteen minutes later, I spoke about "Why are psychiatric drugs the third leading cause of death after heart disease and cancer?" Three psychiatrists out of the over 10,000 at the congress attended and they refused to give interviews and carefully avoided being filmed by the documentary film team that followed me, as if they were on their way to see a porn movie.

The first thing people notice when they start taking a psychiatric drug is its harms. Few people will not experience any harms. The obvious reaction to this would be to tell your doctor that you don't want the drug. But—according to psychiatry's script—your doctor will persuade you to continue, and you will be told that it takes some time before the effect kicks in and that the harms—which doctors call side effects because it sounds nicer—will be less noticeable with time.

So, you carry on. Even when you have become well, which would have happened in most cases, also without drugs, your doctor will insist—according to guidelines based on highly flawed studies that have often been written by doctors on industry payroll[4]—that you need to continue for another number of months, sometimes years, or for the rest of your life.

In their article, "Do antidepressants cure or create abnormal brain states?", Joanna Moncrieff and David Cohen explain why the disease centered model of drug action that assumes that drugs rectify biological abnormalities is incorrect.[52] A drug centered model is far more plausible. In this model, which is not a model but just plain reality, psychotropic drugs create abnormal states that may coincidentally relieve symptoms. Alcohol's disinhibiting effects may relieve symptoms of social phobia, but that doesn't imply that alcohol corrects a chemical imbalance underlying social phobia.

The authors argue that a disease-based model—as insulin for diabetes—could be considered established if:

- the pathology of psychiatric conditions or symptoms had been delineated independently from the characterization of drug action, and drug action could be extrapolated from that pathology;

- rating scales used to evaluate drug treatment in clinical trials reliably detected changes in the manifestations of an underlying disease process rather than detecting drug-induced effects;

- animal models of psychiatric conditions selected specific drugs;

- drugs thought to have a specific action in certain conditions were shown to be superior to drugs thought to have nonspecific effects;

- healthy volunteers showed different or absent patterns of effects, compared with diagnosed patients, since drugs would be expected to exert their therapeutic effects only in an abnormal nervous system;

- and the widespread use of supposedly disease-specific drugs led to demonstrable improvements in short- or long-term outcome of psychiatric disorders.

None of this is true for psychiatric drugs. In a circular chain of logic, the monoamine theory of depression was formulated primarily in response to observations that the first marketed depression pills increased brain monoamine levels. Monoamines include serotonin, dopamine, and norepinephrine, but there is no evidence that there is a monoamine abnormality in depression. The depression rating scales, e.g. the Hamilton scale,[53] contain items that are not specific to depression, including sleeping difficulties, anxiety, agitation, and somatic complaints. These symptoms are likely to respond to the nonspecific sedative effects that occur with many depression pills and other substances, e.g. alcohol, opium and psychosis pills, which could then also be considered depression pills, but we do not prescribe alcohol or morphine for people with depression or call them depression pills.

Using the Hamilton scale, even stimulants like cocaine, ecstasy, amphetamine, and ADHD drugs could be considered depression pills. Almost everything could. Indeed, many drugs that are not considered to be depression pills show comparable effects to them, e.g. sleeping pills, opiates, stimulants, and some psychosis pills.[52]

Recent sharp increases in depression pill use have been accompanied by increased prevalence and duration of depressive episodes and rising levels of sickness absence.[52] In all countries where this relationship has been examined, the increased use of psychiatric drugs has been accompanied by an increase in disability pensions for mental health reasons.[3] This shows that psychiatric drugs are harmful.

---

1. We should all contribute to changing psychiatry's seriously misleading narrative.

2. Depression pill is the correct term for an "antidepressant", as it makes no promises.

3. Major tranquillizer is the correct term for an "antipsychotic", as this is what the drug does, to patients, healthy volunteers, and animals. It may also be called a psychosis pill, which makes no promises.

4. Sedative is the correct term for an "anti-anxiety" drug, as this is what the drug does, to patients, healthy volunteers, and animals.

5. Speed-on-prescription is the correct term for ADHD drugs, as they work like amphetamine, and as some of them are amphetamine.

6. "Mood stabilizer" is like the unicorn. Since such a drug doesn't exist, the term should not be used.

Flawed Trials Have Led the Psychiatrists Astray

The rating scales used in placebo-controlled trials of psychiatric drugs for measuring the reduction of symptoms have made the psychiatrists believe that the drugs work and that the effect is specific for the disorder being treated. However, such results do not say anything about whether the patients have been cured or can live a reasonably normal life.

Furthermore, the effects measured with these scales are unreliable. Virtually every single placebo-controlled drug trial in psychiatry is flawed.[4,54]

Since the trials are flawed, systematic reviews of trials are also flawed, and guidelines are flawed. Even the drug approval process is flawed. The drug regulators don't pay enough attention to the flaws. They don't even ask the drug companies for the many missing data or appendices which, according to the indexes the companies provide, should have been included in their applications.[55]

Cold Turkey in the Placebo Group

In the vast majority of the trials, the patients were already on a drug similar to the one being tested against placebo. After a short washout period without this drug, the patients are randomized to the new drug or placebo. There are three main problems with this design.

First, the patients who are recruited for the trials are those who have not reacted too negatively on getting such a drug before.[52] They will likely therefore not react negatively to the new drug, which means that the trials will underestimate the harms of psychiatric drugs.

Second, when patients who have tolerated a psychiatric drug are randomized to placebo, they will likely react more negatively to this than if they had not been in treatment before. This is because psychiatric drugs have a range of effects, some of which can be perceived as positive, e.g. euphoria or emotional numbing.

Third, the cold turkey that some patients in the placebo group go through harms them. It is therefore not surprising that the new drug seems to be better than placebo. Introducing longer washout periods does not remove this problem. If people have been permanently brain damaged before entering the trials, washout periods cannot compensate, and even if that is not the case, they could suffer from withdrawal symptoms for months or years.[7,56,57]

Thousands of trials of psychosis pills (antipsychotics) have been carried out, but when my research group recently searched for placebo-controlled trials in psychosis that only included patients who had not received such a drug earlier, we found only one trial.[58] It was from China and appeared to be fraudulent. Thus, all placebo-controlled, randomized trials of psychosis pills in patients with schizophrenia spectrum disorders were flawed, which means that the use of psychosis pills cannot be justified based on the evidence we currently have.[4]

The first trial that was not flawed was published on 20 March 2020,[59] 70 years after the discovery of the first psychosis pill, chlorpromazine, that Rhône-Poulenc marketed in 1953 with the trade name Largactil, which means broad activity.

However, even 70 years wasn't enough for the psychiatrists to come to their senses. They were not yet ready to draw the consequences of their results, which their abstract demonstrates:[59]

> "...group differences were small and clinically trivial, indicating that treatment with placebo medication was no less effective than conventional antipsychotic treatment (Mean Difference = -0.2, 2-sided 95% confidence interval -7.5 to 7.0... p = 0.95). Within the context of a specialised early intervention service, and with a short duration of untreated psychosis, the immediate introduction of antipsychotic medication may not be required for all cases of first episode psychosis in order to see functional improvement. However, this finding can only be generalised to a very small proportion of FEP [first episode psychosis] cases at this stage, and a larger trial is required to clarify whether antipsychotic-free treatment can be recommended for specific subgroups of those with FEP."

I have translated what this means for those of us who do not have guild interests to defend:

> Our study was small, but it is unique because it only included patients who had not been treated with a psychosis pill before. We found that psychosis pills are not needed for patients with untreated psychosis. This is great progress for patients, as these drugs are highly toxic and make it difficult for them to come back to a normal life. Based on the totality of the evidence we have, the use of psychosis pills in psychosis cannot be justified. Psychosis pills should only be used in placebo-controlled randomized trials of drug-naïve patients.

The authors of a 2011 Cochrane systematic review of psychosis pills for early episode schizophrenia pointed out that the available evidence doesn't support a conclusion that the use of such drugs in an acute early episode of schizophrenia is effective.[60] This is one of the very few Cochrane reviews of psychiatric drugs that can be trusted.[4,54] There are huge problems with most Cochrane reviews, e.g. Cochrane reviews in schizophrenia routinely include trials in a meta-analysis (which is a statistical summary of the results of several trials) where half of the data are missing.[4] This is garbage in, garbage out, with a nice little Cochrane logo on it, as Tom Jefferson said in an interview in the article, "Cochrane—a sinking ship?"[61]

To find out for how long patients should be advised to continue taking their drugs, so-called maintenance studies, also called withdrawal studies, have been carried out. These studies are highly misleading because of cold turkey effects. A large meta-analysis of 65 placebo-controlled trials found that only three patients needed to be treated with psychosis pills to prevent one relapse after one year.[62] This looks very impressive, but the result is totally unreliable. The apparent benefit of continued treatment with psychosis pills decreased over time and was close to zero after three years. Thus, what was seen after one year was iatrogenic harm, which was described as a benefit.

When follow-up is longer than three years, it turns out that discontinuing psychosis pills is best. There is only one appropriately planned and conducted maintenance trial, from Holland. It has seven years follow-up, and patients who had their dosages decreased or discontinued fared much better than those who continued taking psychosis pills: 21 of 52 (40%) versus 9 of 51 (18%) had recovered from their first episode of schizophrenia.[63]

Leading psychiatrists interpret the maintenance studies of psychosis pills and depression pills to mean that these drugs are highly effective at preventing new episodes of psychosis and depression, respectively,[4] and that the patients should therefore continue taking the drugs for years or even for life.

Danish researchers tried to repeat the Dutch study, but their trial was abandoned because the patients were scared about what would happen if they did not continue taking their drugs. A psychiatrist involved with the failed trial told me about another, recent withdrawal trial, carried out in Hong Kong.[64] The researchers treated first-episode patients with Seroquel (quetiapine) for two years; discontinued the treatment in half of the patients by introducing placebo; and reported the results at ten years. They found that a poor clinical outcome occurred in 35 (39%) of 89 patients in the discontinuation group and in only 19 (21%) of 89 patients in the maintenance treatment group.

I immediately suspected that the trial was flawed, as this result was the exact opposite of the Dutch result, and that they had tapered off the psychosis pill far too quickly and had caused a cold turkey. As there was nothing about their tapering scheme in the article, I looked up an earlier publication, of the results at three years.[65] They didn't taper at all; all patients randomized to placebo were exposed to a cold turkey.

The ten-year report was highly revealing: "A post-hoc analysis suggested that the adverse consequences of early discontinuation were mediated in part through early relapse during the 1-year period following medication discontinuation."[64]

The investigators defined a poor outcome as a composite of persistent psychotic symptoms, a requirement for clozapine (Clozaril or Leponex) treatment, or death by suicide. They called their trial double-blind, but it is impossible to maintain the blind in a trial with cold turkey symptoms, and it is highly subjective whether there are any psychotic symptoms and whether clozapine should be given. I'm much more interested in whether the patients return to a normal life, and a table showed that after ten years, 69% of those who continued taking their drug were employed versus 71% in the cold turkey group, a quite remarkable result considering the iatrogenic harms inflicted on the latter group.

I consider this trial highly unethical because some patients commit suicide when they experience cold turkey effects. Robert Whitaker has demonstrated that this trial design is lethal.[1,66] One in every 145 patients who entered the trials for risperidone (Risperdal, Janssen), olanzapine (Zyprexa, Eli Lilly), quetiapine (Seroquel, AstraZeneca) and sertindole (Serdolect, Lundbeck) died, but none of these deaths were mentioned in the scientific literature, and the FDA didn't require them to be mentioned. The suicide rate in these clinical trials was 2-5 times higher than the norm.

It is no wonder that AstraZeneca that sells Seroquel was happy to fund a trial in Hong Kong that was seriously flawed in favour of their drug.[64]

The investigators' attempt at explaining away what they found is breathtaking. They wrote that their result in the third year raised the suggestion that, "there might be a time window or critical period during which a relapse might be course-modifying." The plausibility of the existence of such a time window between year two and three is zero. As it is highly variable when or if a patient relapses, there cannot exist any such time window. The psychiatrists deliberately harmed half of their patients, but they concluded they did nothing wrong and that their patients, or their disease, or a "time window" are to blame.

Lack of Blinding

Because of the conspicuous side effects of psychiatric drugs, trials labeled double-blind are not double-blind. Quite a few patients—and their doctors—know who is on drug and who is on placebo.[4] When a trial is not adequately blinded, the small differences recorded can be explained purely by bias in the outcome assessment on a subjective rating scale.[4]

In trials supposed to be double-blind, investigators may report positive effects that only exist in their imagination. This occurred in a famous trial funded by the US National Institute of Mental Health in 1964, which is still highly cited as evidence that psychosis pills are effective. It was a trial of 344 newly admitted patients with schizophrenia who were randomized to phenothiazines such as chlorpromazine, or to placebo.[67] The investigators reported, without offering any numerical data, that the drugs reduced apathy (indifference) and made movements less retarded, the exact opposite of what these drugs do to people, which the psychiatrists had admitted a decade earlier.[3] The investigators claimed a huge benefit for social participation (effect size of 1.02) and that the drugs make the patients less indifferent to the environment (effect size 0.50). The drugs do the opposite. They also claimed, with no data, that 75% versus 23% were markedly or moderately improved and suggested that the drugs should no longer be called tranquillizers but antischizophrenic drugs. Their study contributed to shaping the erroneous beliefs that schizophrenia can be cured with drugs and that psychosis pills should be taken indefinitely.[1]

Psychosis pills do not have clinically relevant effects on psychosis. Despite the formidable biases—cold turkey, lack of blinding, and industry funding that involves torturing the data till they confess,[4,51]— the published outcomes have been very poor.[4] The least clinically relevant effect corresponds to about 15 points on the Positive and Negative Syndrome Scale (PANSS)[68] commonly used in trials. Yet, what was reported in placebo-controlled trials of recent drugs submitted to the FDA was only 6 points[69] even though scores easily improve when someone is knocked down by a tranquillizer and expresses abnormal ideas less frequently.[9]

Depression pills don't work either. The smallest effect that can be perceived on the Hamilton scale is 5-6,[70] but only about 2 is obtained in flawed trials.[71,72]

Some meta-analyses have found that the effect of depression pills is larger if the patients are severely depressed,[71,73,74] and the pills are generally recommended for severe and sometimes also for moderate depression. However, the reported effects are very small for all depression severities, e.g. 2.7 for patients with a baseline Hamilton score above 23 which is considered very severe depression,[74] and 1.3 for milder degrees.[71] Moreover, it is likely just a mathematical artefact that the effect seems to be slightly larger in severe depression.[75] Since the baseline scores for severe depression are larger than for mild depression, any bias will influence the measured result more in patients with severe depression than in those with mild depression. If we assume that the bias due to insufficient blinding is 10% when estimating the effect in the drug group and, for the simplicity of the example, that there is no bias in the placebo group and no improvement between baseline and the final visit, then a Hamilton baseline score of 25 would still be 25 after treatment. But because of the bias, there would be a 2.5-point difference between drug and placebo. If the baseline is 15, that difference would only be 1.5.

The small effect of depression pills measured in flawed trials disappear if the placebo contains atropine, which has similar side effects as the pills, e.g. dry mouth.[76] Such trials were done many years ago when the depression pills were tricyclics. Many psychiatrists say that these are more effective than newer depression pills (but also more dangerous, which is why they are rarely used). Despite this, the effect in nine trials with atropine in the placebo only corresponded to 1.3 on the Hamilton scale.[76] The "effect" of the newer drugs is around 2.3, or almost double as much.[71,72]

It is very easy to make almost any substance with side effects "work" for depression, including stimulants.[77] Three of the 17 items on the Hamilton scale are about insomnia, and that issue alone can yield six points on the scale,[53] or three times as much as the "effect" in biased trials. And if a person goes from maximum anxiety to no anxiety, eight points can be earned.

Irrelevant Outcomes

What do doctors want to achieve with drugs? Above all, to avoid suicides and deaths from other causes. Moreover, to get the patients back to a normal life, with good social contacts.

Sometimes, this cannot be obtained. Most patients who get a diagnosis of depression live depressing lives, e.g. are married to the wrong person, have a bullying boss, a tedious job, or a chronic disease, and it is hardly the job of doctors to try to get them out of this predicament. Moreover, there are no pills for this, but these people are nonetheless routinely prescribed depresssion pills, which are seen as the "solution" to life's troubles.

A score on a rating scale doesn't tell us whether the patient is well. Over a thousand placebo-controlled trials of depression pills have been carried out, but I have not seen any that measured whether the patients were *cured* by a drug, i.e. whether they came back to a normal productive life. If any such trials existed, we would have known about them. Unless they showed that the drugs made the situation worse and were therefore buried in company archives.[4]

According to the American Psychiatric Association's disease manual, DSM-5, major depression is present when the patient exhibits 5 or more of 9 symptoms that "cause clinically significant distress or impairment in social, occupational, or other important areas of functioning." Given how the disorder is defined, it makes no sense that drug trials don't use these outcomes.

A trial with such outcomes was inappropriate, as it was a withdrawal trial that only told us that the cold turkey harms the psychiatrists inflicted on their patients were bigger for some drugs than for others.[78] Unsurprisingly, patients on Prozac (fluoxetine, the sponsor's, Eli Lilly's product) could endure a short treatment interruption where the patients got placebo because this drug has an active metabolite that remains in the body for a long time. In contrast, a statistically significant increase in harms occurred after missing just one dose of paroxetine (Paxil or Seroxat).

Lilly's trial was grossly unethical. The abstinence symptoms after paroxetine withdrawal were severe, which was expected based on clinical observations and a previous, similar study also sponsored by Lilly.[79] The patients experienced "statistically significantly worsened severity in nausea, unusual dreams, tiredness or fatigue, irritability, unstable or rapidly changing mood, difficulty concentrating, muscle aches, feeling tense, chills, trouble sleeping, agitation and diarrhea during placebo substitution."[78] In Lilly's previous trial,[79] roughly one-third of the patients on paroxetine or sertraline (Zoloft) experienced worsened mood, irritability and agitation, and had an increase in the Hamilton score of at least eight, which is the difference between being mildly depressed and severely depressed.[74]

Lilly sacrificed the patients for a marketing advantage. Many patients suffered from an abstinence depression caused by the cruel trial design, and the various harms they experienced increase the risk of suicide, violence and homicide.[4] This was known long before the trial was carried out.[2,4,80]

It was not surprising at all that, "Patients treated with paroxetine reported statistically significant deterioration in functioning at work, relationships, social activities and overall functioning."[78]

---

1. If you are being asked to participate in a clinical trial with a psychiatric drug, you should investigate very carefully what it is about and whether it is ethically acceptable.

2. Ask the doctor for all documentation, including the full trial protocol and investigator's brochure, which might be the only place where the harms have been listed, also from animal experiments.

3. Pay attention to conflicts of interest. Will the doctor or the department benefit financially from conducting the trial?

4. Will the raw data in anonymized form be made available to the investigators and to independent researchers, allowing them to do their own analyses? Will all patients who ask for these data get them?

5. Ensure you get written confirmation before you make a decision. If the data will not be made available, or your doctor becomes uncomfortable when you ask, you should refuse to participate and publish your experiences as a deterrent for bad research practice and to warn other patients.

Suicides, Other Deaths and Other Serious Harms

It is a well-guarded secret how many people are killed by psychiatric drugs. This has been obscured in many ways.

The easiest way is to wipe the deaths under the carpet, "so that we don't raise concerns," as a Merck scientist was told when he was overruled by his boss.[51] The scientist had judged that a woman on Merck's arthritis drug Vioxx (rofecoxib) had died from a heart attack, but the cause of death was changed to unknown, also in Merck's report to the FDA. Other sudden cardiac deaths on Vioxx disappeared before the trial results were published. When the many deaths could no longer be hidden, Merck withdrew Vioxx, in 2004. I have estimated that Vioxx killed around 200,000 people, most of whom had not even needed the drug.[51]

Fraud with lethal consequences is common in drug trials,[4,51] and our major medical journals, in this case the *New England Journal of Medicine*, often willingly contribute to it by publishing flawed trials and by not taking action when action is clearly needed in order to save patients' lives.[51]

Psychiatry is no exception. Only about half the suicides and other deaths that occur in psychiatric drug trials are published.[81]

Another big problem is cold turkey in the placebo group. Since virtually all trials suffer from this design defect, they will underestimate how deadly psychiatric drugs are.

Psychosis Pills

Psychosis pills are very toxic and likely the deadliest of all psychiatric drugs.[4] When I wanted to find out how deadly they are, I decided to focus on elderly, demented patients. I assumed that few of them would be in treatment before they were randomized and that there would be enough patients to draw a conclusion because many of them die, whether they are on drugs or not.

I found a meta-analysis of placebo-controlled trials in dementia with a total of about 5,000 patients.[82] After only ten weeks, 3.5% had died while they were on one of the newer psychosis pills, olanzapine (Zyprexa), risperidone (Risperdal), quetiapine (Seroquel) or aripiprazole (Abilify), while 2.3% had died on placebo. Thus, for every 100 people treated for ten weeks, one patient was killed with a psychosis pill. *This is an extremely high death rate for a drug.*

Since half of the deaths are missing, on average, in published research,[81] I looked up the corresponding FDA data based on the same drugs and trials. As expected, some deaths had been omitted from the publications, and the death rates were now 4.5% versus 2.6%, which means that psychosis pills kill two patients in a hundred in just ten weeks.[83]

I also found a Finnish study of 70,718 community-dwellers newly diagnosed with Alzheimer's disease, which reported that psychosis pills killed 4-5 people per year compared to patients who were not treated.[84] If the patients received more than one psychosis pill, the risk of death was increased by 57%. As this was not a randomized trial, the results are not fully reliable, but taken together, these data show a death rate so high that I cannot recall having seen another drug the patients don't need that is so deadly.

Should we extrapolate these results to young people with schizo-phrenia? Yes. In evidence-based healthcare, we base our decisions on the best available evidence. This means the most reliable evidence, which are the data just above. Thus, absent other reliable evidence, we will need to assume that psychosis pills are also highly lethal for young people. We should therefore not use psychosis pills for anyone, also because an effect on psychosis has never been demonstrated in reliable trials.

We don't need to go any further, but it might be interesting. According to the FDA, most of the deaths in the demented patients appeared to be either cardiovascular (e.g. heart failure, sudden death) or infectious (e.g. pneumonia).[83] Young people on psychosis pills also often die from cardio-vascular causes and suddenly. And I would expect some of them to die from pneumonia. Psychosis pills and forced admission to a closed ward make people inactive. When they lie still in their bed, the risk of pneumonia increases. Depression pills, sedatives/hypnotics and antiepileptics also increase the risk of pneumonia. Furthermore, a closed psychiatric ward is not a department of internal medicine, and if a patient develops pneumonia while lying zombie-like in a bed, it might not be noticed.

The psychiatrists are fully aware—and have often written about it—that the lifespan for patients with schizophrenia is 15 years shorter than for other people, but they don't blame their drugs or themselves, but the patients. It is true that these people have unhealthy lifestyles and may abuse other substances, in particular tobacco. But it is also true that some of this is a consequence of the drugs they receive. Some patients say they smoke because it counteracts some of the harms of psychosis pills, which is correct because tobacco increases dopamine while the drugs decrease dopamine.

It is also indisputable that psychosis pills kill some patients with schizophrenia because they can cause huge weight gains, hypertension, and diabetes, but how common is it?

When I tried to find out why young people with schizophrenia die, I faced a roadblock, carefully guarded by the psychiatric guild. It is one of the best kept secrets about psychiatry that the psychiatrists kill many of their patients with psychosis pills. I described my experiences with the roadblock guards in 2017 on the Mad in America website, "Psychiatry ignores an elephant in the room,"[85] but subsequent events were even worse.

Large cohort studies of people with a first-episode psychosis provide a unique opportunity for finding out why people die. However, as there is too little information in these studies, or no information at all, about the causes of death, you need to ask.

The TIPS Study: 12% of the Patients Died in Just 10 Years

In 2012, Wenche ten Velden Hegelstad and 16 colleagues published 10-year follow-up data for 281 patients with a first-episode psychosis (the TIPS study).[86] Although their average age at entry into the study was only 29 years, 31 patients (12%) died in less than 10 years. However, the authors' detailed article was about recovery and symptom scores.

They took no interest whatsoever in all these deaths, which appeared in a flowchart of patients lost to follow-up and were not commented upon anywhere in their paper.

In the text, they mentioned only 28 deaths (11%), so it was not even clear how many died. In March 2017, I wrote to Hegelstad and inquired about the causes of death. Most patients were still on psychosis pills 10 years after they started, which I considered very frightening because around half of them would have developed tardive dyskinesia (a terrible movement disorder, which is often irreversible but masked by ongoing treatment) and because many, if not all, would have developed permanent brain damage at this point.

I sent a reminder ten days later and was told I would get an answer shortly. Two months later, I wrote again and mentioned that it was important for the world to know what all these young patients had died from. I also asked if we needed to file a Freedom of Information request to get this information.

Hegelstad replied that they were preparing a manuscript detailing the information I asked for. The paper came out the next month, in *World Psychiatry*, but the number of deaths was now different from their first paper, and the information I had requested wasn't there.[87]

Two months later, Robert Whitaker and I wrote to the editor of *World Psychiatry*, professor Mario Maj, asking for his help in getting a unique insight into why so many patients had died so young. We hoped he would ensure that the knowledge the investigators had in their files became public by publishing our short letter to the editor and by asking them to respond. "That would be a great service to psychiatry, the patients, and everyone else with an interest in this vitally important issue."

We explained in our letter that the authors had reported that 16 patients died by suicide, 7 by accidental overdoses or other accidents, and 8 from physical illnesses, including 3 from cardiovascular illness:

> "In order to attempt to separate iatrogenic causes of death from deaths caused by the disorder, we need to know: When did the suicides occur? Suicides often occur early, after the patients have left hospital,[88] and are sometimes iatrogenic. A Danish register study of 2,429 suicides showed that, compared to people who had not received any psychiatric treatment in the preceding year, the adjusted rate ratio for suicide was 44 for people who had been admitted to a psychiatric hospital.[89] Such patients would of course be expected to be at greatest risk of suicide because they were more ill than the others (confounding by indication), but the findings were robust and most of the potential biases in the study were actually conservative, i.e. favoured the null hypothesis of there being no relationship. An accompanying editorial noted that there is little doubt that suicide is related to both stigma and trauma and that it is entirely plausible that the stigma and trauma inherent in psychiatric treatment—particularly if involuntary— might cause suicide.[90]
>
> What does accidental overdoses and other accidents mean? Did the doctors overdose or did the patients overdose themselves by mistake, and which types of accidents were involved? Psychotropic drugs can lead to falls, which can be fatal, and suicides are sometimes miscoded as accidents.[91]
>
> It is surprising that 8 young people died from physical illness. What were these illnesses exactly and what were the cardiovascular illnesses? If some of these people suddenly dropped dead, it could be because antipsychotics can cause QT prolongation."

Eight days later, we were told by Maj that, "Unfortunately, although it is an interesting piece, it does not compete successfully for one of the slots we have available in the journal for letters."

So, there was no space in the journal for our letter of 346 words, no longer than a journal abstract, and no interest in helping young people survive by finding out what kills them at such a young age. This was psychiatry at its worst, protecting itself while literally killing the patients.

Five days later, I appealed Maj's decision:

> "Allow me to add that people I have talked to in several countries about deaths in young people with schizophrenia—psychiatrists, forensic experts and patients—have all agreed that we desperately need the kind of information we asked you to ensure we get from the very valuable cohort of patients Melle et al. reported on in your journal.
>
> There is widespread and well-substantiated suspicion that the reason we have not seen a detailed account of causes of death in cohorts like the one in the TIPS study by Melle et al. published in your journal is that the psychiatrists prioritise protecting their guild interests rather than protecting the patients. By declining to publish our letter and get the data out that Melle et al. have in their files, you contribute to that suspicion. We previously asked one of the investigators, Wenche ten Velden Hegelstad, to provide us with these data but were told on 10 May this year that they would be published... They have not been published, as what Melle et al. have published in your journal is not an adequate account of why these young people died.
>
> Therefore, we call on you to ensure these data get out in the open, for the benefit of the patients. We believe it is your professional and ethical duty—both as a journal editor and as a doctor—to make this happen. This is not a matter about the slots you have available in the journal for letters. It is a matter of prioritization."

We did not hear from Maj again.

In contrast to the authors of the TIPS study, Danish psychiatry professor Merete Nordentoft was forthcoming when I asked her about the causes of death for 33 patients after 10 years of follow-up in the OPUS study, also of patients with a first-episode psychosis.[92] I specifically mentioned that suicides, accidents and sudden unexplained deaths could be drug related. Nordentoft sent a list of the deaths and explained that the reason cardiac deaths were not on the list was probably because the patients had died so young. In the death certificates, she had seen some patients who had simply dropped dead, one of them while sitting in a chair.

This is how it should be. Openness is needed if we want to reduce the many deaths that occur in young mental health patients, but very few psychiatrists are similarly open as Nordentoft. I asked Hegelstad about the conflicting numbers of deaths and also asked to get details on the causes of death. I didn't hear from Hegelstad again.

TIPS was supported by grants from 15 funders, including the Norwegian Research Council, the US National Institute of Mental Health, three drug companies (Janssen-Cilag, Eli Lilly and Lundbeck), and other funders in Norway, Denmark, and USA. I asked all the funders for detailed information on the deaths, emphasizing that funders have an ethical obligation to ensure that information of great importance for public health, which has been collected in a funded study, gets published.

The silence was daunting. In December 2017, the Norwegian Research Council published its policy about making research data accessible for other researchers, which left no doubt that this should happen, without delay, and not later than when the researchers published their research.[93]

Janssen-Cilag replied: "We find the data on mortality published by Melle et al. 2017 in *World Psychiatry* fully satisfactory." Both they and Eli Lilly encouraged us to contact the authors, which was absurd, as I had written to the companies that the authors had refused to share their data with us. Lundbeck did not reply.

Five months after I had written to the Norwegian Research Council, I received a letter from Ingrid Melle who had been asked by the council to respond to me. I was told I had misread Figure 1 in the original paper[86] where I had counted 49 deaths. I hadn't. Their figure is seriously misleading because flowcharts otherwise always show numbers of patients who were lost or died during a study. I have redrawn the figure here:

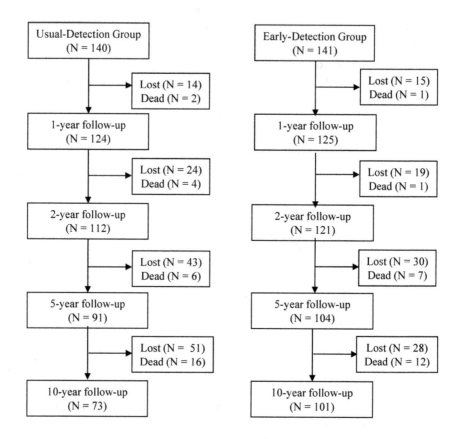

Fig. 2-1: Overview of Patient Participation in a Long-Term Follow-Up Study of Early Detection in Psychosis

The reason that there were 31 deaths, and not 28, in Melle's paper was because they had added 1-3 years of observation time, which didn't exactly make it more transparent what the researchers had been doing.

Melle sent me a table, which was not particularly informative (see Table 2-1 on next page).

Melle explained that accidental drug overdose means taking too much of an illegal substance, or substance, or too strong a substance by accident, and that is does not refer to prescription drugs. If information about overdoses was ambiguous, it was defined as probable suicide.

	N	%
Alive	**250**	**89.0**
Suicide	**16**	**6**
Confirmed suicide; violent means	4	1.4
Confirmed suicide; other highly lethal means	5	1.8
Confirmed suicide; drug overdose or other intoxications	2	0.7
Confirmed suicide, other means	2	0.7
Probably suicide; drug overdose or other intoxications	3	1.1
Other causes of death	**15**	**5**
Accidental drug overdose	5	1.8
Accidents	2	0.7
Natural death, cardiovascular illness	3	1.1
Natural death, other illnesses	2	0.7
Natural death of unknown causes	3	1.1

Table 2-1: Causes of Death during the First 10 Years of Treatment

This was really interesting. Why did 16 young people (6%) commit suicide in just 10 years? And why was this vitally important information not explored by the researchers? We cannot conclude it was their schizophrenia that led to suicide. It is more likely the drugs enforced upon them, other forced treatments, involuntary admissions to psychiatric wards, humiliation, stigmatization and loss of hope, e.g. when patients are told that their disease is genetic, or can be seen in a brain scan, or is lifelong, or requires lifelong treatment with psychosis pills. I am not making this up.[4] It all happens, and some patients get it all. It is no wonder they might kill themselves when there is no hope.

The accidental drug overdoses are also of interest. The term is a bit tragicomic because patients with schizophrenia are usually overdosed by their doctors with prescription drugs and if they take an illegal drug as well, it is rarely possible to say that it was the illegal drug that killed them and not the prescription drugs. It could be the combination, and it might not have happened if the patient had not been forced to take psychosis pills and other dangerous drugs, e.g. depression pills and antiepileptics, both of which double the risk of suicide (see Chapter 1).

Finally, there were eight deaths from "natural causes." It is not natural for a young person to die. I would have liked to know in detail what happened. It might be "natural" for psychiatrists that young people die in psychiatry but that's because the psychiatrists ignore their own role in this.

I wrote again to the Norwegian Research Council, pointing out that Melle had told me that the data on causes of death contained the full information available to the doctors writing out the death certificates. I

requested to see this information, in an anonymized format. I also
noted that psychosis pills had been used liberally in the study and that
some or all the deaths could have potentially been caused by the drugs
the patients were on, which often involve taking many drugs. I found it
curious, considering the very high death rate of 12% (see Table 2-1 on
p. 45), that the authors had not discussed whether the deaths could
have been caused by the drugs and had not reported which drugs the
patients were on.

Finally, I noted that Melle had asked me: "Since you are writing
with a Nordic Cochrane Centre letterhead, I'm curious if Cochrane has
any plans for doing anything in this area?" I noted that I did not
understand the relevance of this question. Why would I *not* use the
letterhead for my own center?

I heard no more. But Melle's inappropriate comment about my
center's letterhead, which I used in all official correspondence, seems to
have been part of a concerted effort with the aim of removing me from
my job as Cochrane director.[36]

Harassments from Psychiatrists and Cochrane

In my letter to the 15 funders, the final paragraph was

> "You may consider this a Freedom of Information request,
> which means that if your organisation does not have detailed
> information on the deaths in the TIPS study, we expect your
> organisation to obtain this information from Hegelstad and to
> send it to us. Anything short of this would be unethical in our
> view, and we are convinced that patients with psychotic
> disorders agree with us (I am Protector for the Hearing Voices
> Network in Denmark)."

This would seem straightforward, but the US Stanley Medical
Research Institute did not write to me. Instead, psychiatrist Edwin
Fuller Torrey, associate director of research at the institute, complained
about me in two letters to the CEO of the Cochrane Collaboration,
journalist Mark Wilson, where he, among other things, wrote:[36]

> The Cochrane Collaboration's credibility rests upon the
> assumption of objectivity... Such objectivity appears to be very
> much in doubt for Dr. Peter C. Gøtzsche who identifies himself
> as the Director of the Nordic Cochrane Center and as the
> Protector of the Hearing Voices Network in Denmark. This
> organization promotes the belief that auditory hallucinations

are merely one end of a normal behavioral spectrum, thus casting doubt on whether schizophrenia actually exists as a disease, and that hearing voices are caused by trauma in childhood, for which there is no solid evidence. Given such clear lack of objectivity, I personally would not find any Cochrane publication on mental illness to be credible.

Torrey also wrote that the Hearing Voices Network encourages people who take psychosis pills for their schizophrenia to stop taking their medication, and that, "It is very difficult to imagine how anyone with these views could possibly be objective regarding a Cochrane study of antipsychotics, thus impugning your credibility which is your most important asset."

This was bizarre. How can my objectivity be "very much in doubt" when I merely ask for the number of deaths and their causes? Furthermore, contrary to Torrey's assertions, there is solid evidence that psychosis is related to childhood traumas, with a clear dose-response relationship.[29,30]

Torrey also drew the logically false conclusion that because I am protector of the Hearing Voices Network, no Cochrane publication on mental illness is credible. There is no relation between these two things. Here is an excerpt of a comment the Network sent to me:

> We take issue with Torrey's attempts to discredit the Hearing Voices Movement to add leverage in his attempt to discredit Professor Peter Gøtzsche. In 2016, we invited Gøtzsche to be protector because of his pioneering work regarding psychiatric research. We are honored to have him as our protector.
>
> We believe that Torrey's comments to Mr. Wilson regarding Gøtzsche being our protector to be bordering on the ridiculous when he attempts to discredit the whole Cochrane Collaboration.
>
> We would ask that Torrey stops using the network as a platform to insult a respected professor along with the Cochrane Collaboration. We would also suggest that he considers apologizing for his disrespectful remarks about voice hearers.

The motto of the Cochrane Collaboration is "Trusted evidence," which Wilson had demanded we should all use, also in our letterheads, as if we were a drug company and not an independent scientific organisation registered as a charity. He also required we used short names for our centres, which created great confusion among journalists who often wrote the "Cochrane Nordic Centre" even though my centre's name was the "Nordic Cochrane Centre:"

Trusted evidence. Informed decisions. Better health.

Cochrane
Nordic

Nordic Cochrane Centre
Rigshospitalet, Dept. 7811
Blegdamsvej 9
2100 Copenhagen Ø, Denmark
Tel: +45 35 45 71 12
E-mail: general@cochrane.dk
www.nordic.cochrane.org

Cochrane's motto is highly misleading when it comes to its reviews of psychiatric drugs. As I have explained above, very few of them can be trusted.

My criticism of the drug industry's organized crime,[4,51] psychiatric drug trials and the overuse of psychiatric drugs was never popular at Cochrane headquarters after Wilson took office in 2012 and changed an idealistic grassroots movement into a business with a focus on brand and sales.[36] Wilson and his deputy's harassments of me were particularly damaging after I published the article about ten myths in psychiatry that are harmful for the patients in 2014,[38] and when I explained in a major journal in 2015 why long-term treatment with psychiatric drugs causes more harm than good.[36,94]

Wilson also bullied me on this occasion. Instead of dismissing Torrey's complaint, which was the only right thing to do, Wilson wrote to me that I had broken Cochrane's Spokesperson Policy by using my center's letterhead and my title and that this would reasonably lead any reader to assume that the request was from the Nordic Cochrane Centre and that the views expressed were those of the center. Wilson wanted to apologize to Torrey for "any confusion in this regard." Quite interesting, that one bully wanted to apologize to the other bully when the person between the bullies had done nothing wrong.

The setup was ridiculous, and even Cochrane's own hired lawyer didn't find I had broken the policy, neither in this case, nor in another similar case that was also about psychiatry,[36] but such trifles don't matter for bullies. There was no problem, but Wilson invented one. It was clear that the request came from the center; that I as Director was authorized to speak on behalf of my center; and my views were even shared by my staff. Furthermore, my letter was not a public announcement, but a letter to a funder. No one could become "confused."

US lawyer Ryan Horath described the farce this way:[36]

> Cochrane leaders became obsessed about Gøtzsche using Nordic Cochrane letterhead to send this request. And a very large number of people seem to agree with the board's obsession... JESUS CHRIST, WHAT IS WRONG WITH YOU PEOPLE? A researcher is making inquiries about the suppression of information regarding children who died in a clinical trial and everyone is worried about what letterhead it is written on?... Even worse, it is clear the outrage over use of Cochrane letterhead is feigned outrage, as this was a private letter. Was Fuller Torrey confused about whether the letter represented Cochrane's views? Apparently not... Instead, Torrey argued that Gøtzsche was not 'objective' and this damaged Cochrane's reputation—something totally different... So, Cochrane leadership's use of this complaint in its case was misleading. The complaint is about one thing, and they used it as evidence of another (false allegation). That is how kangaroo courts operate.

What Is the Bottom Line of Psychosis Pills?

Countless unreliable studies have been concocted to fabricate a fairytale about psychosis pills helping people survive their psychosis. I have dissected some of them in my previous book.[4] They have serious flaws and the patients that are being compared—those on psychosis pills and those not—are not comparable to begin with. Particularly a Finnish doctor, Jari Tiihonen, has published one misleading study after the other.[4]

Don't pay any attention to these reports. Whitaker once wrote to me that it requires extraordinary mental gymnastics by the psychiatrists to conclude that these drugs, which cause obesity, metabolic dysfunction, diabetes, tardive dyskinesia, lethal cardiac arrhythmias, and so on, protect against death. Furthermore, as noted above, the psychiatrists often take away the patients' hope of one day living a normal life. Why bother about having a healthy lifestyle if life will never be worth living? It is not only psychosis pills, often in combination with many other psychiatric drugs, that kill the patients, it is the whole package psychiatry delivers to them.

If acutely disturbed patients need something to calm them down, benzodiazepines (sleeping pills) are far less dangerous and even seem to work better.[95] When I have asked patients if they would prefer a benzodiazepine or a psychosis pill next time they developed a psychosis and felt they needed a drug, all of them have said they preferred a benzodiazepine. Why don't they get it then?

1. Do everything you can to avoid getting treated with a psychosis pill.

2. Do everything you can to avoid anyone dear you to get treated with a psychosis pill.

3. If a doctor insists, give the doctor a copy of my book and say you will sue, if the doctor ignores you.

4. Ensure you can document that you warned the doctor, e.g. by recording the conversation, bringing a journalist to the meeting, or demanding a written note from the doctor on the spot, not later. If doctors get in trouble, they often deny what happened, and they might even change the written records.[45]

Depression Pills

Depression pills are the poster child for psychiatry, the pills we hear most about, and the pills which are most used, in some countries by more than 10% of the population.

As noted, it is one of psychiatry's best kept secrets that the psychiatrists kill many patients with psychosis pills. Another well-kept secret is that they also kill many patients with depression pills, e.g. elderly patients who lose balance and break their hip.[4,96]

The psychiatrists have fought really hard to hide the terrible truth that depression pills double the risk of suicide, not only in children but also in adults.[2,4,97-100] The placebo-controlled trials are hugely misleading in this respect, and a lot has been written about how drug companies have hidden suicidal thoughts, suicidal behavior, suicide attempts and suicides in their published trial reports, either by wiping the events under the carpet for no one to see, or by calling them something else.[2,4,101] This massive fraud is routine in drug companies. I devoted a huge part to the fraud in my 2015 psychiatry book,[4] and shall therefore only mention some recent research results here.

My research group found that, compared to placebo, depression pills double the occurrence of FDA defined precursor events for suicide and violence in healthy adult volunteers;[97] that they increase aggression in children and adolescents 2-3 times,[55] a very important finding considering the many school shootings where the killers were on depression pills; and that they increase the risk of suicide and violence by 4-5 times in middle-aged women with stress urinary incontinence, judged by FDA defined precursor events.[98] Furthermore, twice as many women experienced a core or potential psychotic event.[98]

Psychiatrists dismiss research results that go against their interests. They have also criticized our use of precursor events, but there is nothing wrong with this. Using precursor events to suicide and violence is similar to using prognostic factors for heart disease. As smoking and inactivity increase the risk of heart attacks, we recommend people to stop smoking and to start exercising.

It is cruel that most psychiatric leaders say—even on national TV[102]—that depression pills can be given safely to children because there wasn't a statistically significant increase in suicides in the trials, only in suicidal thoughts and behavior, as if there is no relation between the two.[4] The psychiatrists reward the companies for their fraud while they sacrifice the children. We all know that a suicide starts with suicidal thinking followed by preparations and one or more attempts.

A US psychiatrist who argued that suicidal behavior should not count because it is "an unvalidated, inappropriate surrogate" contradicted himself, as he wrote in the same paper that, "A history of a prior suicide attempt is one of the strongest predictors of completed suicide," and also wrote that the rate of suicide is 30 times greater in previous attempters than in non-attempters.[103] This is full-blown cognitive dissonance with deadly consequences for our children.

When I wrote my 2015 book, it became clear to me that suicides must be increased not only in children, but also in adults, but the many analyses and reports were confusing with some having found this and others not.[4]

The crux of the matter is that many suicide attempts and suicides are left out in reports. In 2019, I found additional evidence of this, when I compared a trial publication[104] with the corresponding 1008-page clinical study report submitted to drug regulators.[105] The authors of the published report did not mention that two of 48 children on fluoxetine (Prozac) attempted suicide versus none of 48 children on placebo. The internal study report of another placebo-controlled trial of fluoxetine given to children and adolescents also showed that many events that increase the risk of suicide were not reported in Lilly's publications in medical journals.[106]

Suicide attempts and suicides are not only concealed during the trial. Most often, they are also omitted when they occur just after the randomized phase is over.[4] When the FDA did a meta-analysis of sertralineused in adults (Table 30 in their report),[107] they did not find an increase in suicide, suicide attempt or self-harm combined, risk ratio 0.87, 95% confidence interval 0.31 to 2.48 (see Table 2-2).

Pfizer's own meta-analysis found a halving of the suicidal events when all events that occurred later than 24 hours after the randomized phase stopped were omitted.[108] However, when Pfizer included events occurring up to 30 days later, there was an increase in suicidality events of about 50%.

		sertraline		placebo			
	Follow-up	n	N	n	N		RR (95% CI)
FDA 2006[107]	24 hours	7	6,950	7	6,047	0.87	(0.31 to 2.48)
Pfizer 2009[108]	24 hours	5	6,561	8	5,480	0.52	(0.17 to 1.59)
Pfizer 2009[108]	30 days	25	10,917	14	9,006	1.47	(0.77 to 2.83)
Gunnel 2005[109]	> 24 hours	24	7,169	8	5,108	2.14	(0.96 to 4.75)

Table 2-2: Sertraline Trials in Adults

Key: *n:* number of suicides and suicide attempts; *N:* number of patients; *follow-up:* time after the randomized phase ended; *RR:* risk ratio; *CI:* confidence interval.

A 2005 meta-analysis conducted by independent researchers using UK drug regulator data found a doubling in suicide or self-harm when events after 24 hours were included (see table).[109] These researchers noted that the companies had underreported the suicide risk in their trials, and they also found that nonfatal self-harm and suicidality were seriously underreported compared to reported suicides.

Another meta-analysis carried out in 2005 by independent researchers of the published trials was very large, as it included all drugs (87,650 patients) and all ages.[110] It found double as many suicide attempts on drug than on placebo, odds ratio (which is the same as risk ratio when events are rare) 2.28, 95% CI 1.14 to 4.55. The investigators reported that many suicide attempts must have been missing. Some of the trial investigators had responded to them that there were suicide attempts they had not reported, while others replied that they didn't even look for them. Further, events occurring shortly after active treatment was stopped were not counted.

The reason it is so important to include suicidal events that occur after the randomized phase is over is that it reflects much better what happens in real life rather than in a tightly controlled trial where the investigators motivate the patients to take every single dose of the trial drug. In real life, patients miss doses because they forget to take the pills to work, school or a weekend stay, or they introduce a drug holiday because the pills have prevented them from having sex (see below).

It differs from trial to trial what happens when it is over. Sometimes, the patients are offered active treatment, sometimes only the treated patients continue with active treatment, and sometimes there is no treatment.

In 2019, two European researchers finally put an end to the psychiatrists' fierce denial that depression pills are also dangerous for adults. They re-analyzed FDA data and included harms occurring during follow-up.[99] They were criticized and published additional analyses.[100] Like other researchers, they found that suicide events had been manipulated, e.g. two suicides "that occurred during the lead-in phase were incorrectly recorded as placebo suicides."[100] They reported double as many suicides in the active groups than in the placebo groups, odds ratio 2.48 (95% CI 1.13 to 5.44).

There should be no more debate about whether depression pills cause suicides at all ages. They do. Even the FDA, which has done it utmost to protect drug companies marketing depression pills,[2,4] was forced to give in when it admitted in 2007, at least indirectly, that depression pills can cause suicide at any age:[4,111]

> "All patients being treated with antidepressants for any indication should be monitored appropriately and observed closely for clinical worsening, suicidality, and unusual changes in behavior, especially during the initial few months of a course of drug therapy, or at times of dose changes, either increases or decreases. The following symptoms, anxiety, agitation, panic attacks, insomnia, irritability, hostility, aggressiveness, impulsivity, akathisia (psychomotor restlessness), hypomania, and mania, have been reported in adult and pediatric patients being treated with antidepressants... Families and caregivers of patients should be advised to look for the emergence of such

symptoms on a day-to-day basis, since changes may be abrupt."

The FDA finally admitted that depression pills can cause madness at all ages and that the drugs are very dangerous—otherwise daily monitoring wouldn't be needed. It needs to be said, however, that daily monitoring is a fake fix of a deadly drug problem. People cannot be monitored every minute, and many have killed themselves with violent means, e.g. hanging, shooting, stabbing or jumping in front of a train, shortly after they seemed to be perfectly fine to their loved ones.[2,4]

But the organized denial continues undeterred.[4] Two years after FDA's announcement, the Australian government stated: "The term suicidality covers suicidal ideation (serious thoughts about taking one's own life), suicide plans and suicide attempts. People who experience suicidal ideation and make suicide plans are at increased risk of suicide attempts, and people who experience all forms of suicidal thoughts and behaviours are at greater risk of completing suicide."[112]

True, but why did suicidality not include suicide? If you want to find out how dangerous mountaineering is, and you include injuries when people have serious thoughts about climbing mountains and attend a fitness center, and injuries when they plan to climb a mountain and when they attempt to do so, would you then exclude deaths due to falls? Of course, you wouldn't, but this was what the Australian government did. They showed the lifetime prevalence of suicidality, divided into suicidal ideation, suicide plan and suicide attempt, but there were no data on suicides.[112]

There is a long way to go. In our review of 39 popular websites in 10 countries, which we published in 2020, we found that 25 stated that depression pills may cause increased suicidal ideation, but 23 (92%) of them contained incorrect information, and only two (5%) websites noted that the suicide risk is increased in people of all ages.[32]

Depression pills can cause violence and homicide.[2,4] But this is also one of psychiatry's well-guarded secrets. Particularly in the USA, psychiatrists and authorities won't tell the public if the perpetrator was on a depression pill. It can take a long time and involve Freedom of Information requests or lawsuits before anything gets revealed.

It took quite a while before we learned that the Germanwings Flight 9525 pilot that took a whole plane with him when he committed suicide in the Alps, and that the Belgian bus driver who killed many children by driving his bus into a wall, also in the Alps, were on a depression pill.

Even though we suspected serious underreporting of harms in the clinical study reports we examined—some outcomes appeared only in individual patient listings in appendices, which we had for only 32 of our 70 trials, and we didn't have case report forms for any of the trials—we found alarming events, which you will never see in publications in medical journals.[55] Here are some examples:

- Four deaths were misreported by the company, in all cases favoring the active drug.

- A patient receiving venlafaxine (Effexor) attempted suicide by strangulation without forewarning and died five days later in hospital. Although the suicide attempt occurred on day 21 out of the 56 days of randomized treatment, the death was called a post-study event as it occurred in hospital and treatment had been discontinued because of the suicide attempt.

- Although patient narratives or individual patient listings showed they were suicide attempts, 27 of 62 such attempts were coded as emotional lability or worsening depression, which is what you see in publications, not the suicide attempts.

- One suicide attempt (intentional overdose with paracetamol in a patient on fluoxetine) was described in the adverse events tables as "elevated liver enzymes," which is what you get if you drink too much alcohol.

It is of particular relevance for the many school shootings that the following events for 11 patients on a depression pill were listed under aggression in patient narratives for serious adverse events: homicidal threat, homicidal ideation, assault, sexual molestation, a threat to take a gun to school, damage to property, punching household items, aggressive assault, verbally abusive and aggressive threats, and belligerence.

Akathisia is a horrible feeling of inner restlessness, which increases the risk of suicide, violence, and homicide. We could only identify akathisia if we had access to the verbatim terms, but we nonetheless found that, like aggression, akathisia was seen double as often on the pills than on placebo. In three sertraline (Zoloft) trials where we had access to both the verbatim and the coded preferred terms, akathisia was coded as "hyperkinesia," and miscoding seemed to have been prevalent also in trials of paroxetine (Paxil or Seroxat) since we didn't find a single case of akathisia.

For Eli Lilly's drugs, fluoxetine (Prozac) and duloxetine (Cymbalta), we compared our findings with the summary trial reports that are available on the company's website.

In most cases, adverse events were only shown if they occurred in, for example, at least 5% of the patients. In this way, the companies may avoid reporting many serious harms. We found that suicidal events and harms increasing the risk of violence were seriously under-reported:

Only 2 of 20 suicide attempts (17 on drug, 3 on placebo) were documented. None of 14 suicidal ideation events (11 vs 3) were mentioned. Only 3 akathisia events (15 vs 2) were mentioned.

Akathisia is also seen with other psychiatric drugs, e.g. psychosis pills (see below). Akathisia is Greek and means inability of sitting still. The patients may behave in an agitated manner, which they cannot control, and they can experience unbearable rage, delusions, and disassociation.[80] They may endlessly pace, fidget in their chairs, and wring their hands—which have been described as actions that reflect an inner torment.[1] Akathisia need not have visible symptoms but can be extreme inner anxiety and restlessness, which is how this harm is described in the product information for Zyprexa. In one study, 79% of mentally ill patients who had tried to kill themselves suffered from akathisia.[1] Another study reported that half of all fights at a psychiatric ward were related to akathisia,[5,113] and a third study found that moderate to high doses of haloperidol (Haldol), a psychosis pill, made half the patients markedly more aggressive, sometimes to the point of wanting to kill their psychiatrists.[1]

Since depression pills have purely symptomatic effects and many harms, it is highly relevant to find out what the patients think about them when they weigh the benefits against the harms. They do this when deciding whether to continue in a trial till the end or to drop out of it.

It was huge work to study dropouts in the placebo-controlled trials. We included 71 clinical study reports we had obtained from the European and UK medical agencies, which had information on 73 trials and 18,426 patients. No one, apart from my research group, had ever read the 67,319 pages about these trials before, which amount to 7 m if stacked. But it was well worth the effort; 12% more patients dropped out while on drug than while on placebo.[114]

This is a terribly important result. The psychiatrists' view is that depression pills do more good than harm,[4] and the patients' view is the opposite. The patients preferred placebo even though some of them were harmed by cold turkey effects. That means that the drugs are even worse than found in the cold turkey trials.

Because we had access to detailed data, we could include patients in our analyses that the investigators had excluded, e.g. because some measurements had not been made. Our result is unique and reliable, in contrast to previous reviews using mostly published data. They failed to find more dropouts on drugs than on placebo,[114] e.g. a large review of 40 trials (6391 patients) reported that dropouts were the same (relative risk 0.99) when paroxetine was compared with placebo.

Next, we decided to look at quality of life in the same trials. Given our result for dropouts; the tiny benefit of depression pills that lacks any relevance for the patients; and the pills' many and frequent harms, we expected that quality of life would be worse on pills than on placebo.

We were perhaps a bit naïve, because we had now come too close to the secrets of depression pills. What we found—or rather didn't find— was shocking.[115] The reporting of health-related quality of life was virtually non-existent. In five trials, it was unclear which instrument was used and no results were available. We included 15 trials (4,717 patients and 19,015 pages of study reports), a substantial amount of data on which to base conclusions. However, 9 of the 15 clinical study reports displayed selective reporting, and in the companies' online registers, there was selective reporting for all 15 trials. We received 20 publications from Eli Lilly and 6 from the GlaxoSmithKline register. There was selective reporting in 24 of the 26 publications. Despite this extensive selective reporting, we found only small differences between drug and placebo.

This was more than a roadblock; it was sabotage. The companies are obliged to ensure that what they submit to drug regulators to obtain marketing approval is an honest account of what happened, and that important data or information have not been left out. We wondered why the drug regulators had not asked the companies for the missing data.

The Pills that Destroy Your Sex Life are Called Happy Pills

In the upside-down world of psychiatry, the pills that destroy your sex life are called happy pills. Half of the patients who had a normal sex life before they started on a depression pill will have their sex life disturbed or made impossible.[4,116] The sexual disturbances can become permanent and when the patients find out that they will never again be able to have intercourse, e.g. because of impotence, some kill themselves.[117,118] When I lectured for Australian child psychiatrists in 2015, one of them said he knew three teenagers taking depression pills who had attempted suicide because they couldn't get an erection the first time they tried to have sex.

It is so cruel. And yet, the professional denial is widespread. The patients are often humiliated or ignored by their doctors who refuse to believe them. Some patients are told that such complications from taking depression pills are impossible, and others are put on psychosis pills after having been told that their problem is psychosomatic.[118]

One patient who had sent a couple of links to studies and reviews about enduring sexual dysfunction received this reply: "If you wish to have such 'syndrome' continue what you are doing... read obscure studies and reviews in obscure databases and I can guarantee you that you will have it till the end of your life!"

By far most patients who are on a depression pill will feel something has changed in their genitals, and many complain that long after they came off the pills, their emotions continue to be numbed; they also don't care about life or other people like they did before the pills.

Psychiatry professor David Healy has told me that some patients can rub chili paste into their genitals and not feel it. In his work as an expert witness, he has seen data no one outside the drug industry has ever seen, which are sealed as soon as the company settles out of court with the victims. Healy has described that, in some unpublished phase 1 trials, over half of healthy volunteers had severe sexual dysfunction that in some cases lasted after treatment stopped.[119]

The numbness of the genitals is used in marketing. The depression pill Priligy (dapoxetine) has been approved in the European Union for treating premature ejaculation. It is interesting to contrast this with the information provided in package inserts, e.g. for Prozac (fluoxetine).[120] Right from the start, it puts the blame on the patient rather than on the drug: "changes in sexual desire, sexual performance, and sexual satisfaction often occur as manifestations of a psychiatric disorder." Accordingly, an FDA scientist found out that SmithKline Beecham had hidden sexual problems with paroxetine by blaming the patients, e.g. women who could no longer get an orgasm were coded as "Female Genital Disorder."[121]

Healy sent a petition to Guido Rasi, the director of the European Medicines Agency (EMA) in June 2019 signed by a large group of clinicians and researchers. EMA indicated they would ask companies to mention enduring sexual dysfunction in the labels of depression pills. Six months later, Healy sent another letter to Rasi stating that the drug agencies had responded that these conditions might stem from the illness rather than the treatment. He added: "Melancholia, which is very rare, can lead to lowered libido but the kind of depression for which SSRIs [depression pills] are given does not lower libido. Indeed, just like people comfort eat when they have 'nerves' so they often have more sex in an attempt to handle their 'depression.'"

In its package insert,[120] Eli Lilly stated that, "some evidence suggests that SSRIs can cause such untoward sexual experiences." *Some* evidence? No. When you look at *all* the evidence, it becomes abundantly clear that these drugs ruin people's sex lives.

Lilly's denial mode continues: "Reliable estimates of the incidence and severity of untoward experiences involving sexual desire, performance, and satisfaction are difficult to obtain, however, in part because patients and physicians may be reluctant to discuss them." Since we have this evidence, what is then the problem Lilly has in acknowledging what it shows?

In Lilly's trials,[120] "decreased libido was the only sexual side effect reported by at least 2% of patients taking fluoxetine (4% fluoxetine, <1% placebo)." If you don't ask, you won't see the problems. In a carefully conducted study, 57% of 1022 people who had a normal sex life before they came on a depression pill experienced decreased libido; 57% had delayed orgasm or ejaculation; 46% no orgasm or ejaculation; and 31% had erectile dysfunction or decreased vaginal lubrication.[116] There was nothing about this in Lilly's package insert apart from: "There have been spontaneous reports in women taking fluoxetine of orgasmic dysfunction, including anorgasmia. There are no adequate and well-controlled studies examining sexual dysfunction with fluoxetine treatment. Symptoms of sexual dysfunction occasionally persist after discontinuation of fluoxetine treatment."

Some package inserts are more truthful, e.g. for venlafaxine (Effexor):[122] decreased libido 2%, abnormal ejaculation/orgasm 12%, impotence 6%, and orgasm disturbance 2%. But this is still far from the truth.

1. If you feel depressed, don't go to your doctor who will very likely prescribe a depression pill for you.

2. Never accept treatment with a depression pill. It is likely to make your life more miserable.

3. Don't believe anything doctors tell you about depression pills. It is highly likely to be wrong.

4. Depression pills are dangerous. They increase the risk of suicide, violence and homicide at all ages.

5. Depression pills are likely to destroy your sex life, in the worst case permanently.

6. Consult a psychotherapist. You might also consider if you need a social worker, counsellor, or lawyer.

Lithium

Lithium is a highly toxic metal used for bipolar disorder. Like most other psychiatric drugs, it sedates people and renders them inactive. Serum concentrations must be closely monitored because toxicity can occur at doses close to therapeutic concentrations.

In package inserts, patients and their families are warned that the patient must discontinue lithium therapy and contact the doctor if they experience diarrhea, vomiting, tremor, mild ataxia (not explained even though few patients know that it means loss of control over bodily movements), drowsiness, or muscular weakness.

The risk of lithium toxicity is increased in patients with renal or cardiovascular disease, severe debilitation or dehydration, or sodium depletion, and for patients receiving medications that may affect kidney function, e.g. some antihypertensives, diuretics and pain-relieving arthritis drugs. Very many drugs can change serum levels of lithium, which is therefore very difficult to use safely, and the list of serious harms is long and frigthening.[123]

Psychiatrists praise this highly dangerous drug, saying it works and prevents suicide. However, the psychiatrists that reviewed lithium in 2013 concluded cautiously.[124] There were six suicides in the trials, all on placebo, but the authors noted that the existence of just one or two moderately sized trials with neutral or negative results could materially change their finding. Selective reporting of deaths is always an issue, particularly with old trials, and most of the trials are old. Furthermore, patients were often titrated to the most appropriate dose before half of them were abruptly put on placebo, which increases the risk of suicide and violence.

A Swedish psychiatrist and I therefore did our own meta-analysis excluding the cold turkey trials. We found only four trials. There were three suicides in the placebo groups, and nine versus two deaths in favor of lithium, but because of the small numbers and unreliable data (about half of all deaths are missing in psychiatric drug trials),[81] we did not draw any firm conclusions.[125]

Does lithium help? I am reluctant to use the four trials we found to answer that question. They had highly subjective outcomes, such as if the patients had relapsed or had improved by a certain amount, and the trials must have been poorly blinded because the side effects of lithium are very pronounced.

If we want to know what lithium does to people, we need large trials with something in the placebo that gives side effects so that it is more difficult to break the blinding, and there should be long follow-up after the randomized phase is over where the patients are slowly tapered off lithium, so that we can see what the long-terms harms are. We already know that lithium can cause irreversible brain damage.[123]

This is not a drug I would recommend to anyone.

Antiepileptic Pills

As already noted, antiepileptics double the risk of suicide.[126] Psychiatrists use them a lot, but like most other drugs used in psychiatry, their main effect is to suppress emotional responsiveness by numbing and sedating people.[56]

Also like most other psychiatric drugs, they are used for virtually everything. I have seen many patients entering the door of psychiatry with a variety of "starting diagnoses," all ending up being prescribed a gruesome cocktail of drugs that included antiepileptics.

I am not surprised that psychiatrists think antiepileptics "work" for mania, because anything that knocks people down and incapacitates them seems to "work" for mania. But it is nothing else than a chemical straitjacket.

Antiepileptics not only sedate people, they can also do the opposite and make them manic.[126] Depression pills can also make people manic,[122] but this is not desirable, as it usually leads to a cascade of additional, dangerous drugs like psychosis pills and lithium that increase the risk of dying and make it very difficult for the patients to return to a normal life. Furthermore, the patients are now called bipolar even though they suffer from a drug harm.

Drugs for epilepsy have many other harmful effects, e.g. 1 in 14 patients on gabapentin (Neurontin) develops ataxia, which, as just explained, is a lack of voluntary coordination of muscle movements.

Psychiatrists call these horrible drugs "mood stabilizers," which is not what they do, and they never clarified the precise meaning of this term.[9] I googled *mood stabilizers meaning*: "Mood stabilizers are psychiatric medications that help control swings between depression and mania... commonly used to treat people with bipolar mood disorder and sometimes people with schizoaffective disorder and borderline personality disorder." Well, they are used for a lot else, and virtually every psychiatric "career" patient gets them. Just below the Google post, I could read that mood stabilizers not only include antiepileptics and lithium, but also asenapine (Saphris or Sycrest), which is a psychosis pill. Thus, mood stabilizer seems to be a flexible plus term. They forgot to mention alcohol and cannabis, perhaps because they are not prescription drugs, and therefore have no commercial interest for the drug industry.

I have often encountered patients who are on the antiepileptic, lamotrigine (Lamictal). Only two positive trials were published for this drug, while seven large, negative trials were not.[127] Two positive trials are all it takes for FDA approval and the agency regards the others as failed trials, even though we see a failed drug. You need to have a vivid fantasy to imagine what goes on at drug agencies, and the length to which they are willing to go to accommodate the interests of the drug industry.[51] The bottom-line is that drug regulation doesn't work. If it did, our prescription drugs would not be the third leading cause of death,[128-138] and our psychiatric drugs would not have come close to record.[4]

The amount of fraud in the clinical trials in this area is massive.[4] You should not believe anything you read. Forget about these drugs unless you have epilepsy and if you are on them, find help getting off them as quickly as you can.

Pills for the Social Construct Called ADHD

I have never heard about a psychiatric drug that is mainly used short term. All of them, even benzodiazepines, are used for years in most patients, and drugs for the social construct called ADHD are no exception (see pp. 71-74).

These drugs are stimulants and work like amphetamine; in fact, some of them *are* amphetamine. The way the WHO describes them is interesting.[139] Under the heading "Management of substance abuse: amphetamine-type stimulants," they say:

"Amphetamine-type stimulants (ATS) refer to a group of drugs whose principal members include amphetamine and methamphetamine. However, a range of other substances also fall into this group, such as methcathinone, fenetylline, ephedrine, pseudoephedrine, methylphenidate and MDMA or 'Ecstasy'—an amphetamine-type derivative with hallucinogenic properties. The use of ATS is a global and growing phenomenon and in recent years, there has been a pronounced increase in the production and use of ATS worldwide. Over the past decade, abuse of amphetamine-type stimulants (ATS) has infiltrated its way into the mainstream culture in certain countries. Younger people in particular seem to possess a skewed sense of safety about the substances believing rather erroneously that the substances are safe and benign... the present situation warrants immediate attention." Indeed, but what about stimulants on prescription?

Crystal meth is the common name for crystal methamphetamine, a strong and highly addictive drug. In 2017, about 0.6% of the US population reported using methamphetamine in the past year.[140] The usage of stimulants on prescription was 0.8% of the Danish population, also in 2017.

Why then, does the WHO not mention with one word that the increasing use of stimulants on prescription is also a huge problem? Why this double standard?

There were 10,333 drug overdose deaths in USA in 2017 involving stimulants,[140] compared to only 1,378 in 2007.

Meth is regarded as particularly dangerous. We don't know how many people are killed by stimulants on prescription, but we do know that children on these drugs have suddenly dropped dead in the classroom.

We also know that stimulants increase the risk of violence,[129] which is not surprising, given their pharmacological effects. But psychiatrists say the opposite. I have heard them argue many times, also at a hearing in the Danish Parliament, that Ritalin (methylphenidate) protects against crime, delinquency, and substance abuse. This is not true—if anything, they do the contrary.[142]

Like for other psychiatric drugs, the long-term effects are harmful.[4] This was demonstrated in the large US MTA trial that randomized 579 children and reported results after 3, 6, 8 and 16 years.[142-146] After 16 years, those who consistently took their pills were 5 cm shorter than those who took very little, and there were many other harms.[146] We can only speculate which permanent effects these drugs might have on the children's developing brains.

The short-term effect is that the drugs may cause children to sit still in class, but that effect disappears quite quickly. Short-term harms include tics, twitches, and other behaviors consistent with obsessive compulsive symptoms, all of which can become quite common.[9,147] Stimulants reduce overall spontaneous mental and behavioral activity, including social interest, which leads to apathy or indifference, and many children—more than half in some studies—develop depression and compulsive, meaningless behaviors.[56,148]

Animal studies have confirmed this,[148] and we have documented other harms, e.g. that the drugs impair reproduction even after the animals were taken off them.[149]

At school, the compulsive behavior is often misinterpreted as an improvement even though the child may just obsessively copy everything shown on the board without learning anything. Some children develop mania or other psychoses,[56,150] and the harms of the drugs are often mistaken for a worsening of the social construct called a "neurodevelopmental disease," which leads to additional diagnoses, e.g. depression, obsessive compulsive disorder or bipolar—and additional drugs, leading to chronicity.[148]

Trials of ADHD drugs are biased to an exceptional degree, even by psychiatric standards, and therefore most systematic reviews of the trials are also highly biased. A Cochrane review of methylphenidate for adults was so bad that the criticism we and others raised led to its withdrawal from the Cochrane Library.[151] Two Cochrane reviews performed by my former employees, who paid sufficient attention to the flaws, found that every single trial ever performed was at high risk of bias.[152,153]

We also found that the reporting of harms is extremely unreliable.[153] In the British drug agency's review, "psychosis/ mania" was reported to occur in 3% of patients treated with methylphenidate and in 1% of those on placebo. The 3% estimate is 30 times higher than the 0.1% risk of "new psychotic or manic symptoms" that the FDA's Prescribing Information warns about. We also encountered discrepancies within the regulatory documents. In the British drug agency's Public Assessment Report, the rate of aggression for those on methylphenidate was reported to occur in 1.2% on page 61 and in 11.9% on page 63, based on the same population and follow-up time.[153] We furthermore observed huge differences across trials that could not be explained by trial design or patient populations, e.g. decreased libido on methylphenidate was experienced by 11% in one trial versus only 1% in a pooled analysis of three other trials. As quality of life was measured in 11 trials but only reported in 5, where a tiny effect was found,[153] it is reasonable to assume that quality of life worsens on ADHD drugs, which is also what the kids experience. They don't like the drugs.

Doing the right thing in psychiatry is difficult. An Irish child psychiatrist told me he was suspended because he didn't put his children on psychiatric drugs, including ADHD drugs.

Instead of changing our children's brains, we should change their environment. We should also change the psychiatrists' brains so they no longer want to drug children with speed on prescription; perhaps "psychoeducation" would help? ADHD medications are prescribed much more to children of parents with low-skilled jobs, compared with children of more educated parents.[154] These drugs are used as a form of social control, just as psychosis pills are.

A British documentary was very revealing about what is needed. It showed highly disturbing children, which were so difficult to deal with that even critical psychiatrists might conclude that ADHD drugs were necessary. "We cannot have children hanging around in the curtains," as a child psychiatrist told me at a hearing in Parliament about the drugging of children. However, the families got help from psychologists and it turned out that the children were disturbed, which was why they were disturbing. One mother who always reprimanded her "impossible" daughter was taught to praise her instead, and somewhat later, she had developed into a very nice child that was no longer hostile towards her mother.

Sexual abuse of children is frighteningly common and hugely damaging. You can easily find references on the Internet to the fact that about one in ten children have been sexually abused before their 18th birthday. If a child behaves badly, is provocative and defiant, this can easily lead to a diagnosis of ADHD or borderline personality disorder, although it is a reaction to a horrible situation of ongoing sexual abuse that the child doesn't dare talk about to anyone.

One of my colleagues, child psychiatrist Sami Timimi, often asks parents who want him to drug their child for ADHD:[54] "Imagine this drug working perfectly; what changes are you hoping will result from this?" That question may surprise parents, but it is important to say no more until one of them breaks the silence and starts talking about what changes they imagine will happen. That helps Timimi understand the parents' specific areas of concern. Is it, for example, behavior at home, peer relationships, academic performance at school, a lack of a sense of danger? Timimi might then respond that no drug in the world can alter these things in their child. Drugs don't make decisions, have dreams and ambitions, or perform actions.

By discovering the specifics of what the parents want to see change, Timimi can divert their interest from drugs to more targeted measures such as developing parental management skills for children who are more "intense" than most. He helps them understand the anxieties and stress their children may be feeling, or he supports them getting more structured interventions in schools. He also reminds parents that one thing is certain about children: they change as they grow older and often the problems labelled as ADHD (particularly the hyperactivity and impulsivity) tend to diminish and go away as the child matures during adolescence.

Since ADHD is just a label and not a brain disease, we would expect more of those children born in December to get an ADHD diagnosis and be in drug treatment than those born in January in the same class, as they have had 11 fewer months to develop their brains. A Canadian study of one million school children confirmed this.[155] The prevalence of children in treatment increased pretty much linearly from January to December, and 50% more of those born in December were in drug treatment.

The ADHD diagnosis should not be a prerequisite for getting extra help or money for schools, which it is now. It drives the prevalence of this diagnosis upwards all the time, and the use of ADHD drugs, too, which was 3.4 times higher in Denmark in 2017 than in 2007, an increase of 240%.

Some countries have experienced a spiraling increase in the use of psychiatric drugs in children that is directly attributable to school partnerships with hospitals. In one Canadian province, the hospitals aggressively lobbied special services personnel and high school guidance counsellors, who in turn referred any child under stress to the psychiatric department within the children's hospital. The school board hired a school psychiatrist who consulted with staff on school refusal situations and behavioral issues and recommended depression pills or ADHD drugs.

Schools and hospitals have become dangerous places for children and adolescents. How sad this is. Schools should stimulate children, not pacify them with speed on prescription.

> 1. Don't ever accept that your child be treated with speed on prescription.
>
> 2. Don't ever accept this yourself but resist becoming a faceless number in the new market for adults.
>
> 3. Approach children with patience and empathy that allow them to grow up and mature, without drugs.
>
> 4. Work on changing the mechanisms that label more and more children with a psychiatric disorder; they must be able to get the help they need without getting a diagnosis first.

The Final Nails in the Coffin of Biological Psychiatry

When I discuss the state of psychiatry with critical psychiatrists, psychologists and pharmacists I collaborate with, we sometimes ask each other: "Who are most mad, on average, the psychiatrists or their patients?"

This is not as farfetched or rhetorical question as it may seem. When I googled *delusion*, the first entry was from an Oxford dictionary: "An idiosyncratic belief or impression maintained despite being contradicted by reality or rational argument, typically as a symptom of mental disorder."

As you have already seen, right from the start of Chapter 1, and will see more of in the following, the whole of psychiatry is characterized by exactly this. The psychiatrists' predominant idiosyncratic beliefs are not shared by people considered sane, i.e. the general public, but the psychiatrists forcefully maintain them, even when reality, including the most reliable science we have, and rational argument clearly show that their basic beliefs are wrong.

If psychiatry had been a business, it would have gone bankrupt, so let's conclude instead that it is morally and scientifically bankrupt.

One definition of madness is doing the same thing again and again expecting a different result. When a drug doesn't seem to work so well, which is most of the time, psychiatrists increase the dose, change to another drug from the same class, add another drug from the same class, or add a drug from another class.

The science tells us very clearly that these maneuvers will not benefit the patients. Switching drugs, adding drugs or increasing the dose do not result in better outcomes.[156-158] What is certain is that increasing the total dose or number of drugs will increase the occurrence of serious harms, including irreversible brain damage, suicides and other deaths.[4,159,160] Psychosis pills shrink the brain in a dose-dependent manner; in contrast, the severity of the illness has minimal or no effect.[160]

There is no reliable evidence that the psychosis per se can damage the brain.[161] The same applies to other psychiatric disorders, but psychiatrists often lie to their patients telling them that their disease might harm their brains if they do not take psychiatric drugs. Psychiatry professor Poul Videbech wrote in 2014 that depression doubles the risk of dementia,[162] but the meta-analysis he cited did not mention with one word which treatments the patients had received.[163] Other studies indicate that it is the drugs that make people demented.[164,165]

It is routine everywhere to increase the dose, even when the patient has become better. An often-heard comment at conferences at psychiatric wards is: "The patient is doing well after two weeks on Zyprexa, so I will double the dose." This routine is both insane and harmful. The psychiatrist cannot know if the patient might have improved more without Zyprexa. The doctors mislead themselves and their patients all the time based on their misleading "clinical experience" and their treatment rituals go directly against the science.

In this way, many patients end up on terribly harmful drug cocktails they might never escape from. Although it's hard to believe, it's getting worse. A US study of office-based psychiatry found that the number of psychotropic medications prescribed increased markedly, in just nine years up to 2006: visits with three or more medications doubled, from 17% to 33%.[166] Prescriptions for two or more drugs from the same class also increased, although this shouldn't happen.

I was once invited to follow the chief psychiatrist during one day at a closed ward. We talked with several patients. One of them appeared totally normal and reasonable to me, but to my big surprise, the psychiatrist asked me afterwards if I could see that he was delusional. As I couldn't, he explained the patient was delusional because he had been on the Internet and had found out that psychosis pills are dangerous. I replied that they are indeed dangerous and that there is nothing delusional in believing this. I was so stunned that I said no more.

On another occasion, I phoned a psychiatric department in Copenhagen that has a very bad reputation because of the patients the psychiatrists have killed there with their drugs.[45] A desperate patient in great distress had rung me, but it wasn't possible for me to get through to a psychiatrist, although I am a colleague, and it was within normal working hours. I insisted that I needed to talk to someone and was transferred to a head nurse. She told me not to become involved because the patient was delusional. When I asked in what way, she said he had found out that psychosis pills were dangerous. I asked her if she knew whom she was talking to. Oh yes, she knew about me.

I shall now illustrate more of the absurd, delusional world of psychiatry with some examples.

One of my psychiatrist friends sent a letter to a family doctor about a 21-year-old student, recently discharged from a private hospital after she had been given 21 TCMS. When I asked what this is, my friend replied: "Trans-Cranial Magnetic Stimulation, the latest in a long line of crackpot fads to hit psychiatry, designed to separate the worried well from their money."

When she became increasingly anxious, she was given 12 electroshocks. She had two diagnoses, borderline personality disorder and bipolar affective disorder, and was discharged on these drugs (*prn*: as needed; *bd*: twice daily). See Table 2-3.

Drug	Type of drug
diazepam to 20 mg/day	sleeping pill (hypnotic/sedative)
fluvoxamine 300 mg/day	depression pill
mirtazapine 45 mg in the evening	depression pill
quetiapine 400 mg in the evening	psychosis pill
quetiapine to 600 mg/day prn	psychosis pill
aripiprazole 10 mg in the morning	psychosis pill
olanzapine up to 20 mg/day prn	psychosis pill
valproate 1000 mg in the evening	antiepileptic drug
lamotrigine 100 mg bd	antiepileptic drug
topiramate 50 mg bd	antiepileptic drug
lithium 1250 mg/day	"mood stabilizer"

Table 2-3: Medications Dispensed to a 21-Yr-Old Student

This is insane and constitutes gross medical malpractice. No one knows what will happen when all these drugs are given together, only that it is far more dangerous than if fewer drugs are used.

The referral letter notes that the patient sleeps heavily, and her appetite is excessive. She is trying to diet, as she has gained about 50 kg (110 lbs.) with the drugs. She has little energy, interest, or motivation, doesn't exercise or mix socially and has no sexual interest. She has bouts of feeling low and miserable with occasional suicidal ideas due to not liking herself, and also has bouts of feeling "manic," during which she is unpleasantly agitated and tends to overspend in the hope of feeling better.

She also has frequent bouts of agitation and irritability and has described classic akathisia. She has no paranoid ideas; is ritualistic about security and order but there are no true obsessive-compulsive features. She has been anxious since primary school.

My colleague ended his letter by telling the family doctor that this case was a perfect demonstration of why he had published major objections to the standards in mainstream psychiatry. The patient had an anxious personality with secondary depression and did not have borderline personality disorder; apart from this, none of the people using this diagnosis could say what it borders on.

"If she stays on this level of drugs, she will be dead by forty. She is aware of this and wants them reduced but they are all highly addictive and can produce severe withdrawal states, which mimic major mental disorder."

A court case I have been involved with is no different. It is a typical story that illustrates the role of a depression pill as "Psychiatry's Starter Kit."

As far as I can see, this young man should never have been offered a psychiatric drug. He should have been offered psychotherapy for his problems that seemed to be transient. On top of this, he was functioning well when his psychiatrist decided to put him on a depression pill for "depresssion."

His psychiatric "career" lasted 33 years before he finally succeeded to come off the last drug, but he still suffers from long-lasting withdrawal effects. His drug list during all these years is mindblowing. He was prescribed the three main types of psychiatric drugs, sedatives/hypnotics, depression pills and psychosis pills, on and off in various combinations, amounting to a total of three different sedatives/hypnotics, five depression pills and six psychosis pills. He also developed Parkinsonism, likely drug induced, and was treated also for that. Sedatives/hypnotics were prescribed for about 10 years, depression pills for about 25 years, and psychosis pills for about 30 years, and often many drugs at the same time.

It is remarkable that anyone can survive all this and continue being employed.

The psychiatrist stopped the drugs abruptly many times. Not tapering off slowly these drugs after having put a patient on them for long periods of time constitutes highly dangerous malpractice.

I hope he will win the case, but unfortunately, judges are very authoritarian and always emphasize what other psychiatrists do in similar situations. This is wise, as a general precaution, but not when virtually everyone is at fault. If a bank defrauds its customers, it doesn't help in court that other banks do the same. Then why is everyone excused in psychiatry? How will it ever be possible to win cases, given this injustice?

Occasionally, a case is won.[4] Wendy Dolin in Chicago sued Glaxo-SmithKline after her husband, a highly successful lawyer who loved life and had no psychiatric issues, was put on paroxetine because he developed some anxiety regarding work. He got akathisia and threw himself in front of a train six days after starting paroxetine, not realizing it wasn't him that had gone mad; it was the pill that made him mad. Baum & Hedlund in Los Angeles won the case but then? GlaxoSmithKline appealed the verdict.

When Wendy heard I had arranged a meeting about psychiatry in relation to my book launch in 2015,[4] she decided to go to Copenhagen and tell her story. Four other women who had lost a husband, a son, or a daughter to drug induced suicide when there was absolutely no good reason to prescribe a depression pill, also came, on their own account. My program was already full, but I made room for them. This was the most moving part of the whole day. There was stunning silence while they recounted their stories, which can be seen on YouTube.[167]

The colossal use of psychiatric drugs is not evidence-based but is driven by commercial pressures. I studied whether two widely differing drug classes, psychosis pills and depression pills, showed similar patterns in long-term usage. The usage patterns ought to be very different because the main indication for psychosis pills, schizophrenia, has traditionally been perceived as a chronic condition whereas the main indication for depression pills, depression, has been perceived as episodic. However, they were not different. They were the same:[168]

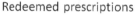

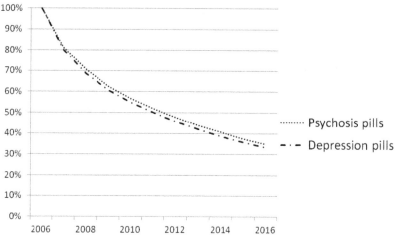

Fig. 2-2: Percentage of Current Users in Denmark Who Redeemed a Prescription for the Same or a Similar Drug in Each of the Following Years After 2006

I started the clock in 2006, following patients onwards in time. That year, 2.0% of the Danish population deemed a prescription for a psychosis pill and 7.3% for a depression pill. Many of the patients had already taken their drug for years, but this group of people also included some who were first-time users in 2006, namely 19.8% vs. 20.0%. This was a remarkably similar percentage for two groups of widely different drugs used for widely different disorders.

The patients got a new prescription every single year till they stopped or came to 2016, my last observation year, when 35% vs 33% of the patients were still on treatment.

These results are shocking. Whatever the flawed guidelines might have tried to tell doctors, they didn't work as expected, and drug usage was clearly not evidence-based. I almost felt I had discovered a new law in nature. Contrary to our hunches, 1 kg (2.2 lbs.) of feathers fall with the same speed as 1 kg (2.2 lbs.) of lead, provided they fall in a vacuum, according to the law of gravity. Similarly, the usage of these two widely different classes of drugs fell with the same speed. A huge proportion of patients continue taking their drug, year in and year out, for more than a decade.

This is iatrogenic harm of epic proportions. The patients dislike the drugs so much that their doctors need to persuade them to take them. Such persuasion is not needed to motivate people to take baby aspirin after a heart attack to reduce the risk of a new attack. Psychosis pills are even forced upon patients against their will "for their own sake." If not forced, few would take them. When healthy people have taken a psychosis pill just to experience what it is like, they have told me, or have published, that they were incapacitated for several days![169] Difficulty reading or concentrating and an inability to work are common harms—but the whole body is affected. We cannot doubt the power of these toxins.

What we are seeing is the result of systematic deception of doctors and patients. The patients are routinely being asked to endure the harms because it may take some time before the drug effect sets in. They are not told that what they perceive as a drug effect is the spontaneous improvement that would have occurred without the drug, or that it can be difficult to come off the drug again. The lie about the chemical imbalance has also contributed. The patients often say that they are afraid of falling ill again if they stop taking their drug because they believe there is something chemically wrong with them.

Mainstream psychiatry doesn't bother about evidence but will continue business as usual pretending my results don't exist saying, "we all know that long-term treatment is good for people; if they don't get their drugs, they will relapse." In 2014, Norwegian psychiatrists wrote about what they called an "alarmingly high discontinuation" rate of psychosis pills in patients with schizophrenia, 74% in 18 months. I would call this a healthy sign, but the psychiatrists argued it highlighted "the clinicians' need to be equipped with treatment strategies that optimize continuous antipsychotic drug treatment."[170] Really? What about forced feeding with pills, like the Strasbourg geese are fed to produce *foie gras*? Psychosis pills make people fat. But psychiatrists don't need to do this. When they don't get their will, or the patients spit out the tablets, they can use depot injections where the drug remains in the body for many weeks.

Next, I decided to find out if there was a similar pattern of usage of benzodiazepines and similar agents (hypnotics/ sedatives), lithium and stimulants (ADHD drugs). Since we have known for decades that benzodiazepines and similar drugs are highly addictive and should only be used for up to four weeks (restricted use was recommended already in 1980 in the UK),[171,172] also because the therapeutic effect disappears quickly, usage of such drugs ought to be very low, and by far most users in a given year should therefore be first-time users. This was not at all the case:[173]

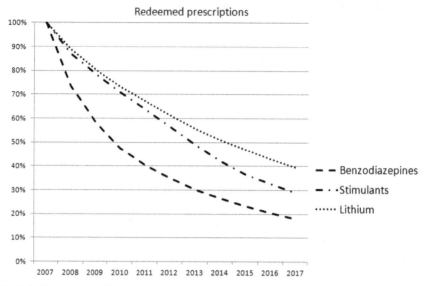

Fig. 2-3: Percentage of Current Users in Denmark Who Redeemed a Prescription for the Same or a Similar Drug in Each of the Following Years After 2007

In 2007, 8.8% of the Danish population redeemed a prescription for a benzodiazepine or similar agent, 0.24% for lithium and 0.16% for a stimulant. For benzodiazepines, only 13.0% were first-time users. For the two other drugs, the numbers were 40.4% and 11.2%, respectively.

The patients got a new prescription every single year till they stopped or came to 2017, my last observation year, when 18%, 29% and 40%, respectively, were still in treatment.

These findings are also disturbing. No matter which psychiatric drug people take or what their problem is, roughly one-third of the patients are still in treatment with the same drug or a similar one ten years later. For benzodiazepines and similar agents, continued use after ten years was "only" 18%, but given what we know about these drugs, it can be argued it should have been zero many years before 2017. This is a disaster. The same can be said about the usage for the other four types of drugs, which was very similar as the span only went from 29% to 40% (see the figures).

If we accept the evidence-based premises that these drugs do not have worthwhile effects, particularly not considering their substantial harms, and that the patients generally dislike them, the data show colossal overuse of the drugs, to a similar degree.

Psychiatry's main focus for the next decades should be on helping patients withdraw slowly and safely from the drugs they are on, instead of telling them that they need to stay on them. But it won't happen. Psychiatry's focus is on itself—a kind of eternal selfie it sends to the world all the time.

Usage of psychiatric drugs continues to increase markedly in virtually all countries. In the UK, psychosis pill prescriptions increased by 5% per year on average and depression pills by 10%, from 1998 to 2010.[174]

In Denmark, the sales of SSRIs (depression pills) increased from a low level in 1992 almost linearly by a factor of 18, closely related to the number of products on the market that increased by a factor of 16 ($r = 0.97$, an almost perfect correlation).[175] This confirms that usage is determined by marketing.

It took almost 30 years after we had the evidence before it became generally accepted that benzodiazepines are addictive.[171] This was expected and should have been investigated from the beginning because their forerunners, the barbiturates, are highly addictive. The first barbiturate, barbital, was introduced in 1903, but it took 50 years before it was accepted that barbiturates are addictive.

Benzodiazepine dependence was documented in 1961 and described in the *British Medical Journal* in 1964. Sixteen years later, the UK Committee on the Review of Medicines published a systematic review of benzodiazepines,[172] concluding that the addiction potential was low, estimating that only 28 persons had become dependent from 1960 to 1977. The fact was that millions had become dependent. In 1988, the Medicines Control Agency finally woke up and wrote to doctors about their concerns.[171]

But the party went on, and history repeated itself. The declining use of benzodiazepines was replaced by a similar increase in the use of depression pills,[175] and a lot of what was previously called anxiety and treated with benzodiazepines was now conveniently called depression.[5] Drug companies, clinicians and authorities denied for decades that depression pills also make people dependent.[171] We did a systematic review of the withdrawal symptoms and found that they were described with similar terms for benzodiazepines and SSRIs and were very similar for 37 of 42 identified symptoms.[176]

Our 2020 study of 39 popular websites from 10 countries was also revealing:[32] 28 websites warned patients about withdrawal effects but

22 stated that SSRIs are not addictive; only one stated that the pills can be addictive and warned that people "may get abstinence symptoms."

Imipramine (Tofranil) came on the market in 1957, and a paper from 1971 describes dependence with this drug when it was tested in six healthy volunteers.[177] As I wrote on the first page in this book, 78% of 2,003 lay people regarded depression pills as addictive in 1991.[178]

Thus, we have known for 50 years or more that depression pills are addictive, and the patients have known it for at least 30 years, but 50 years after we knew it, the dependence problem was still being trivialized by the UK Royal College of Psychiatrists and the National Institute for Health and Care Excellence (NICE),[179] and in the rest of the world, too.

False Information on Withdrawal from UK Psychiatrists

In 2020, I co-authored a paper written by psychology professor John Read, "Why did official accounts of antidepressant withdrawal symptoms differ so much from research findings and patients' experiences?"[179] We noted that the 2018 guidelines from NICE stated that depression pill withdrawal symptoms "are usually mild and self-limiting over about 1 week, but can be severe, particularly if the drug is stopped abruptly," and that guidelines from the American Psychiatric Association asserted that symptoms "typically resolve without specific treatment over 1-2 weeks."

However, a systematic review by James Davies and John Read showed that half of the patients experience withdrawal symptoms; half of those with symptoms experience the most extreme severity rating on offer; and some people experience withdrawal for months or even years.[57] A survey of 580 people reported that in 16% of the patients, the withdrawal symptoms lasted for over 3 years.[57]

In February 2018, Wendy Burn, president of the Royal College of Psychiatrists and David Baldwin, chair of its Psychopharmacology Committee, wrote in *The Times* that, "We know that in the vast majority of patients, any unpleasant symptoms experienced on discontinuing antidepressants have resolved within two weeks of stopping treatment."

Nine clinicians and academics wrote to Burn and Baldwin that their statement was incorrect and had misled the public on an important matter of public safety. We also noted that the College's own survey of over 800 antidepressant users (*Coming Off Antidepressants*) found that withdrawal symptoms were experienced by 63% and lasted for up to 6 weeks, and that a quarter reported anxiety lasting more than 12 weeks. We furthermore noted that within 48 hours of publishing their misleading statement in *The Times*, the College removed the *Coming Off Antidepressants* document from the website.

We asked them to retract their statement or provide supporting research. Baldwin sent two company funded papers with himself as first author. None of them provided data about how long withdrawal symptoms last.

Next, we sent a formal complaint to the College, signed by 30 people, including ten who had experienced withdrawal effects for one to ten years, and ten psychiatrists and eight professors. We noted:

> "People may be misled by the false statement into thinking that it is easy to withdraw and may therefore try to do so too quickly or without support from the prescriber, other professionals or loved ones. Other people, when weighing up the pros and cons of starting antidepressants may make their decision based partly on this wrong information. Of secondary concern is the fact that such irresponsible statements bring the College, the profession of psychiatry (to which some of us belong), and—vicariously—all mental health professionals, into disrepute."

We provided numerous studies and reviews showing the Baldwin-Burn statement to be untrue and asked them to publicly retract, explain and apologize for their misleading statement; provide guidance or training for all the College's spokespersons, including the current president, on the importance of ensuring that public statements are evidence-based and on the limitations of relying on colleagues who are in receipt of payments from the pharmaceutical industry (e.g. Baldwin); and to reinstate, on the College's website, the document *Coming Off Antidepressants*.

The College's registrar, Adrian James, replied that there was "no evidence that the statement in *The Times* was misleading." They dismissed the complaint and James gave four reasons, three of which were either irrelevant or disingenuous. He repeated an earlier claim by Burn that the removal of the survey from their website happened because it was out of date (which it wasn't; it was only six years old). Even when we pointed out that the removal was done within hours after we had shown it includes data contradicting the Baldwin-Burn statement, and that over 50 other items on their website were out of date, but not removed, James adhered to his explanation.

The only relevant comment was that the Baldwin-Burn statement was consistent with NICE recommendations that stated that doctors should advise patients that discontinuation symptoms are "usually mild and self-limiting over about 1 week."

However, James misrepresented the NICE statement by leaving out the next sentence: "but can be severe, particularly if the drug is stopped abruptly."

Four months after *The Times* letter, the CEO of the College, Paul Rees, sent a lengthy reply that merely echoed James. We responded that Rees' emphatic statement, that "it is no part of the College's function to 'police' such debate," implied that even his most senior officials can say anything they like, however false or damaging, and the College would stand by them—as, indeed, it had in this case.

We explained that we were now certain that the Royal College of Psychiatrists prioritizes the interests of the College and the profession it represents over the wellbeing of patients; does not value empirical research studies as the appropriate basis for making public statements and for resolving disputes, and has thereby positioned itself outside the domain of evidence-based medicine; has a complaints process which results in substantive, carefully documented, complaints on serious matters of public safety not being investigated, but rather dismissed out of hand by one individual; has no interest in engaging in meaningful discussion with professional and patient groups who question the College's position on an issue; is prepared to use blatantly disingenuous tactics to try to discredit reasonable complaints, and has thereby positioned itself outside the domain of ethical, professional bodies; is unaware of, or unconcerned about, the distorting influence of the pharmaceutical industry, and the need to maintain a strong, ethical boundary between itself and profit-based organizations.

Even though the College is not accountable to Parliament, or it seems to anyone, we wrote to the Secretary of Health and Social Care and informed the government that,

> "The Royal College of Psychiatrists is currently operating outside the ethical, professional and scientific standards expected of a body representing medical professionals... We believe [the College's] responses show a trail of obfuscation, dishonesty and inability or unwillingness to engage with a concerned group of professionals, scientists and patients.

If a group of scientists and psychiatrists together cannot challenge [the College] in a way that leads to an appropriate, considered response and to productive engagement with the complainants, what hope is there for individual patients to have a complaint taken seriously?"

Burn and Baldwin never retracted their false statement, provided research to support it, or apologized for misleading the public. Neither did James nor Rees ever address our concerns about the complaint procedure.

We made our complaint public, and the BBC's Radio 4 program, *Today*, covered it on 3 October 2018. The College refused to provide a spokesperson to debate with John Read. Instead, Clare Gerada, ex-chair of the Royal College of General Practitioners, represented their perspective. She denigrated the complaint as an "anti-antidepressant story" and vehemently defended the College's official position saying that, "the vast majority of patients that come off antidepressants have no problems whatsoever."

Later, the Royal Society of Medicine launched a podcast series, "RSM Health Matters." The opening topic was about depression pills and withdrawal. One of the two interviewees was Sir Simon Wessely, president of the Royal Society of Medicine (and recent president of the College). The other one was Gerada. None of them disclosed they are married, and both stressed that depression pills enable people to "lead normal lives."

Wessely rejected any link between depression pills and suicide, despite it having been sufficiently well demonstrated for the drugs to carry Black Box Warnings. He also stated, categorically, that depression pills are "not addictive."

Gerada complained that, "Once a year when the prescribing figures come out, we have this soul-searching—why are we prescribing too much of this medication." She said that she personally even prescribes them for people she knows "are going to get depressed" in the future and encouraged "psychiatrists to move away from the fear, which has been propagated I think by the media and certain people, to actually say, is there a space for antidepressants in preventing depression?"

Regarding withdrawal, Gerada stated:

"As a GP [general practitioner] of 26 years... probably 50% of the tens of thousands of patients I have seen have been there with a mental health issue and I can count on one hand the number who have gone on to have long term problems withdrawing from antidepressants or problems coming off antidepressants."

If we interpret "tens of thousands" to mean 30,000, Gerada was talking about roughly 15,000 people with mental health issues. Given her enthusiasm for depression pills, which she uses even "prophylactically," we assumed she prescribed them to 25% of these patients, about 3,750 people. Even if only half of them have ever tried to come off the drugs, then she is claiming an incidence of withdrawal effects of five out of 1,875 or 0.3%. The recent research-based estimate of the actual rate, 56%,[57] is 210 times larger than Gerada's clinical experience.

On November 27, 2018 the BBC Radio program *All in the Mind* invited John Read and psychiatrist Sameer Jauhar to discuss the Davies and Read review. Jauhar explained that, "My hope is that people don't get scared about antidepressants... by thinking that the numbers that have been given out apply to them." When the interviewer asked if patients were warned about withdrawal effects in advance when they started antidepressants, Jauhar replied: "Yes. Like with any other medicine in general medicine you warn patients about any side effects." Read said: "The two largest surveys that we've done, of 1800 and 1400 people, when asked were they ever told anything about withdrawal effects, less than 2% in both surveys said that."[179]

In April 2019, the *Journal of Psychopharmacology* published a critique of the Davies and Read review, which was dismissed as "a partisan narrative." The lead author was Jauhar, accompanied, amongst others, by Baldwin and psychiatrist David Nutt, the journal editor. Three of the six authors, Nutt, Baldwin, and Oxford University psychiatrist Guy Goodwin, disclosed payments from 26 different drug companies, but Jauhar failed to disclose his research funding from Alkermes or his paid lectures for Lundbeck.

The *Journal of Psychopharmacology* is owned by the British Association of Psychopharmacology, which accepts money from the industry in the form of sponsored satellite symposia that are not controlled by the Association. Both the current president, Allan Young, and past presidents, including Nutt, have received money from the drug industry.

John Read's tenacity paid out. On 30 May 2019, the College published a statement where they noted that, "Discontinuation of antidepressants should involve the dosage being tapered or slowly decreased to reduce the risk of distressing symptoms, which may occur over several months... The use of antidepressants should always be underpinned by a discussion about the potential level of benefits and harms, including withdrawal."

Within hours, however, Allan Young, tried to undermine this U-turn by the College. He repeated his drug company line: "So called withdrawal reactions are usually mild to moderate and respond well to simple management. Anxiety about this should not obscure the real benefits of this type of treatment."

In September 2019, Public Health England published a historic 152-page evidence review making important recommendations, including for services to assist people coming off depression pills and other psychiatric drugs, and about better research and more accurate national guidelines.[180] The following month, NICE updated its guidelines in line with the Davies and Read review.

What this illustrates is: We already knew that drug companies don't care about patient safety if it could harm sales.[4,51] We now know that psychiatric leaders also don't care about patient safety if it could threaten their own reputation, the guild they represent, or the flow of money they receive from drug companies. This corruption of a whole medical specialty permeates also our authorities, which rely heavily on specialists when issuing guidelines.

I exposed some of the same people in my 2015 book under the headline: "Silverbacks in the UK exhibit psychiatry's organised denial."[4] It started with my keynote lecture at the opening meeting of the Council for Evidence-based Psychiatry on 30 April 2014 in the House of Lords, chaired by the Earl of Sandwich, "Why the use of psychiatric drugs may be doing more harm than good." The other speakers, psychiatrist Joanna Moncrieff and anthropologist James Davies, gave similar talks.

Two months later, Nutt, Goodwin and three male colleagues bullied me in the first issue of a new journal, *Lancet Psychiatry*.[181]

Their style and arguments revealed the arrogance and blindness at the top of the psychiatric guild everywhere in the world. The title of their paper was: "Attacks on antidepressants: signs of deep-seated stigma?" I was accused, directly or indirectly, of being "anti-psychiatry," "anti-capitalist," having "extreme or alternative political views," launching a "new nadir in irrational polemic," which had suspended my "training in evidence analysis for popular polemic" and made me "prefer anecdote to evidence," which was "insulting to the discipline of psychiatry."

Empty rhetoric this was. What was insulting to psychiatry and to the patients was their article. They claimed that depression pills are among the most effective drugs in the whole of medicine, with an impressive effect on acute depression and on preventing recurrence.

They noted that fewer patients on a depression pill than on placebo drop out of the trials because of treatment inefficacy, which they believed showed that the pills are effective. This is wrong. Many more patients drop out of trials due to adverse events on drug than on placebo.[114] This tends to happen early, and then there are fewer patients who can drop out because of lack of effect in the drug group than in the placebo group. It is therefore a fatal flaw to look at dropouts due to lack of efficacy. We included all dropouts and found that placebo is better than a depression pill.[114]

They mentioned that many people who are not taking depression pills commit suicide, claiming that a "blanket condemnation of anti-depressants by lobby groups and colleagues risks increasing that pro-portion." This is an incredible argument considering that depression pills *cause* suicide!

They claimed that most of those who commit suicide are depressed, but the underlying data don't allow this conclusion.[182] Only about a quarter of people who kill themselves have a diagnosis of depression. Many more get a post-mortem diagnosis based on a so-called psy-chological autopsy. Establishing a diagnosis of a psychiatric disorder in a dead person is a highly bias-prone process. Social acceptability bias threatens the validity of such retrospective diagnosis-making. Relatives often seek socially acceptable explanations and may be unaware of or unwilling to disclose certain problems, particularly those that generate shame or put some of the blame on themselves.

"Some of the safest drugs ever made," they wrote. This is difficult to reconcile with the results of a carefully conducted cohort study that showed that SSRIs kill one of 28 people above 65 years of age treated for one year,[96] and with the fact that the pills double suicides.[97-100]

"The anti-psychiatry movement has revived itself with the recent conspiracy theory that the pharmaceutical industry, in league with psychiatrists, actively plots to create diseases and manufacture drugs no better than placebo." They did not see the irony. It is not a conspiracy theory but a simple fact that psychiatrists have created so many "diseases" that there is at least one for every citizen, and it is also correct that the drugs are not worth using.

The height of professional denial and arrogance came when they suggested that we should ignore "severe experiences to drugs," which they dismissed as anecdotes and claimed might be distorted by the "incentive of litigation." It is deeply insulting to those parents who have lost a child and those spouses who have lost a partner because depression pills drove some people to commit suicide or homicide, or both. In their finishing remarks, the psychiatrists said that my "extreme assertions ... express and reinforce stigma against mental illnesses and the people who have them." It has been documented that it is the psychiatrists that stigmatize the patients, not those who criticize psychiatry.[4]

Sami Timimi is a fellow of the Royal College of Psychiatrists, and he wrote to Burn, its president, in a letter cosigned by 30 people, requesting that the College replace Baldwin as its representative on the Expert Reference Group of Public Health England's Review of Prescribed Medicines, with a College member who is not compromised by conflicts of interest with the pharmaceutical industry. Burn replied that Baldwin's industry involvement did not in any way compromise his work and warned Timimi that he needed to uphold, "the values which the College expects of its members." Like Nutt, Goodwin and other silverbacks, Burn didn't see the irony of her remark. The values seem to allow corruption.

When Scottish psychiatrist Peter Gordon by the end of 2019 expressed his views about psychiatric overmedication and its potential for harm, the chair of the Scottish Division of the Royal College of Psychiatrists made a telephone call to the Associate Medical Director of the NHS Board where Gordon worked and expressed concerns about his mental health.[179] Several of us have experienced to be "diagnosed" by our psychiatric opponents, on my part in a newspaper; during a court case where I was an expert witness;[54] and in a conversation between two psychiatrists at a private party one of my friends overheard.

Another example of fake diagnosis making comes from Emory University in USA where psychiatric professor Charles Nemeroff worked.[4] Millions of drug industry dollars changed hands secretly for more than a decade, and one reason why the scam could continue for so long was that at least 15 whistleblowers were ordered psychiatric evaluations by Emory's psychiatrists who reportedly wrote up such exams without even examining the targeted doctors or gathering factual evidence, where after several of them were fired. Some of these "evaluations" were done by Nemeroff himself. In the Soviet Union, dissidents were given fake psychiatric diagnoses and locked up or disappeared forever.

Such gross ethical transgressions are unique for psychiatry; they are not even possible in other specialties. If a cardiologist loses an academic discussion, or his colleague has exposed his fraud, it won't help him to suddenly claim that his opponent got a heart attack.

Use of Depression Pills for Children Dropped 41%

Here comes a little glimpse of hope in defiance of the dark hole of psychiatry that absorbs all rational thought like dark holes in the universe absorb everything that comes near them.

It is possible to revert the ever-increasing trends in usage of psychiatric drugs if you are similarly tenacious as John Read was in relation to the UK Royal College of Psychiatry.

Due to concerns about the suicide risk, the Danish National Board of Health reminded family doctors in the summer of 2011 that they should not write prescriptions for depression pills for children, which was a task for psychiatrists.[183] At the same time, I began to warn strongly against the suicide risk of the pills. I repeated my warnings countless times in the following years on radio and TV, and in articles, books and lectures. It started with an interview with the managing director of Lundbeck, Ulf Wiinberg, who, in 2011, claimed that depression pills *protect* children against suicide. The interview took place while Lundbeck's US partner, Forest Laboratories, was negotiating compensation with 54 families whose children had committed or attempted suicide under the influence of Lundbeck's depression pills. Elsewhere, I have described Lundbeck's irresponsible behavior, also in relation to a paper I published about the interview.[4]

In Norway and Sweden, there have been no such initiatives. The number of children in treatment increased by 40% in Norway (0-19 years) and 82% in Sweden (0-17 years) from 2010 to 2016, while it decreased by 41% in Denmark (0-19 years) even though professors of psychiatry also in Denmark continued to propagate their false claims that depression pills protect children against suicide.[183]

The Danish National Board of Health had issued several warnings against using depression pills to children before 2011. I therefore believe it is primarily due to my tenacity that the usage went down in

Denmark. I say this to encourage people to fight for a good cause. Despite the formidable odds, it is possible to change things in psychiatry for the better. Not much, but we must not give up the fighting.

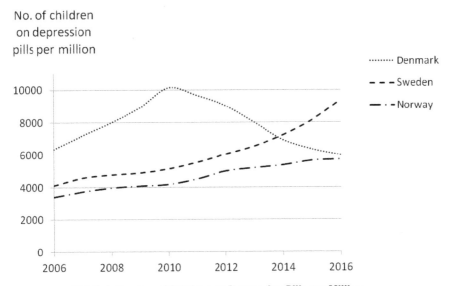

Fig. 2-4: Number of Children on Depression Pills per Million

Number Needed to Treat is Highly Misleading

It is standard in psychiatric research articles to mention the number of patients that need to be treated (NNT) to benefit one of them. The psychiatrists mention NNT all the time as evidence that their drugs are highly effective. But NNT is so misleading that you should ignore everything you read about it.

Technically, NNT is calculated as the inverse of the risk difference (it is actually a benefit difference), and this is simple. If 30% have improved on drug and 20% on placebo, NNT = 1/(0.3-0.2) = 10. Here are the main problems:

First, NNT is derived from seriously flawed trials, with cold turkey in the placebo group, insufficient blinding, and industry sponsorship with data torture and selective publication of the confessions.

Second, NNT only takes those patients into account that have improved by a certain amount. If a similar number of patients have deteriorated, there would be no NNT, as it would be infinite (1 divided by zero is infinite). For example, if a drug is totally useless and only makes the condition after treatment more variable, so that more patients improve and more patients deteriorate than in the placebo group, the drug would seem effective based on NNT because more patients in the drug group would have improved than in the placebo group.

Third, NNT opens the door to additional bias. If the chosen cut-off for improvement does not yield a result the company's marketing department likes, they can try other cut-offs till the data confess. Such manipulations with the data during the statistical analysis, where the prespecified outcomes are changed after company employees have seen the data, are very common.[4,51,101,184] My research group demonstrated this in 2004, by comparing trial protocols we had acquired from ethics review committees with trial publications. Two-thirds of the trials had at least one primary outcome that was changed, introduced, or omitted while 86% of the trialists denied the existence of unreported outcomes (they did not know, of course, that we had access to their protocols when we asked).[184] These serious manipulations were not described in any of the 51 publications.

Fourth, NNT is only about a benefit and completely ignores that drugs have harms, which are much more certain to be experienced than their possible benefits.

Fifth, if benefits and harms are combined in a preference measure, it is not likely that an NNT can be calculated because psychiatric drugs produce more harm than good. In this case, we can only calculate the number needed to harm (NNH). Dropouts during trials of depression pills illustrate this. Since 12% more patients drop out on drug than on placebo,[114] the NNH is 1/0.12, or 8.

The UK silverbacks did not take any of these flaws into account when they claimed that depression pills have an impressive effect on recurrence, with an NNT of around three to prevent one recurrence.[181] It is not surprising that patients want to come back on the drug when their psychiatrists have thrown them into the hell of acute withdrawal by suddenly substituting their drug with placebo. As only two patients are needed to get one with withdrawal symptoms,[57] there cannot exist an NNT to prevent recurrence, only an NNH to harm, which is two.

There cannot exist either an NNT in other depression trials, as the difference between drug and placebo in flawed trials is about 10%,[4] or an NNT of 10, which is far less than the NNH. For example, the NNH for creating sexual problems is less than two for depression pills. Similar arguments and examples can be produced for all psychiatric drugs. Thus, the NNT in psychiatry is bogus. It doesn't exist.

Electroshock

As this book is about drugs, I won't say much about electroshock.[4] Some patients and psychiatrists say it can have a dramatic effect. This could be true, but the average effect is less impressive, and if electroshock were effective, people wouldn't need to receive a long series of shocks, which is usually the case. Furthermore, the shock effect doesn't last beyond the treatment period, and electroshock "works" by causing brain damage, which is scary.[4]

Once, I was asked at a meeting what my view was about a woman who was so depressed that she could hardly be contacted but asked for a glass of water after an electroshock. I said that since this was an anecdote, I would reply with another anecdote. I was once asked to look after a newly admitted man, an unconscious alcoholic. As I needed to rule out meningitis, I tried to insert a needle in his back to tap cerebrospinal fluid for microscopy and culture. It was very difficult to get in and I hit his bone several times. All of a sudden, the drunkard exclaimed loudly: "Bloody hell, stop stinging me in the back!" Had I caused a miracle with my needle and cured the guy? No. Odd things happen all the time in healthcare. Could I have woken up the deeply depressed woman with my needle? Who knows, but why not?

Psychiatrists often say electroshock can be lifesaving, but there is no reliable documentation for this claim whereas we know that electroshock may kill people.[4] Furthermore, it can lead to severe and permanent loss of memory, which leading psychiatrists fiercely deny can happen,[4,23] even though it is well documented that electroshock leads to memory loss in most patients.[4,185-187]

I find it totally unacceptable that electroshock can be enforced upon patients against their will because some patients will die, about 1 per 1000,[186] and others will suffer from serious, irreversible brain damage.[4,23]

---

1. You should not take psychiatric drugs. The only exception I can imagine is a seriously disturbed acute situation where you may need to get some rest and may want a sleeping pill.

2. If you are lucky and have a good psychiatrist who understands the fallibility of psychiatric diagnoses and that drugs or electroshock are not the solution to your problem, continue talking to this doctor.

3. Don't accept electroshock. It is not curative, and some patients are killed or suffer serious and permanent brain damage that reduce their memory and other cognitive functions.

4. If you, after having read all the foregoing, believe psychiatry is evidence-based and that psychiatrists generally know what they are doing, and that you therefore want to consult one you have never met before, I wish you good luck. You will need it.

3   **Psychotherapy**

I know psychiatrists in several countries that don't use psychiatric drugs or electroshock. They handle even the most severely disturbed patients with empathy, psychotherapy, and patience.[1]

The aim of psychological treatments is to change a brain that is not functioning well back towards a more normal state. Psychiatric drugs also change the brain, but they create an artificial third state—an unknown territory—that is neither normal nor the malfunctioning state the patient came from.[2]

This is problematic because you cannot go from the chemically induced third state back to normal unless you taper off the drugs, and even then, it will not always be possible, as you might have developed irreversible brain damage.

A humane approach to emotional pain is very important, and treatment outcomes depend more on therapeutic alliances than on whether psychotherapy or pharmacotherapy is used.[3] Furthermore, the more in agreement physicians and patients are about what is important when being cured from depression, the better the outcomes for positive affect, anxiety and social relationships.[4]

Most of the problems patients face are caused by maladaptive emotion regulation, and psychiatric drugs make matters worse, as their effects constitute maladaptive emotion regulation.[5] In contrast, psychotherapy aims at teaching patients to handle their feelings, thoughts and behavior in better ways. This is called adaptive emotion regulation. It may permanently change patients for the better and make them stronger when facing life's challenges. In accordance with this, meta-analyses have found that the effectiveness of psychotherapy compared with depression pills depend on the length of the trial, and psychotherapy has an enduring effect that clearly outperforms pharmacotherapy in the long run.[6,7]

There are substantial issues to consider when reading reports about trials that have compared psychotherapy with drugs. The trials are not effectively blinded, neither for psychotherapy nor for drugs, and the prevailing belief in the biomedical model would be expected to influence the psychiatrists' behavior during the trial and to bias their outcome assessments in favor of drugs over psychotherapy. Trials that show that the effects of a drug and psychotherapy combined are better than either treatment alone should also be interpreted cautiously, and short-term results are misleading. We should only take long-term results into consideration, e.g. results obtained after a year or more.

I will not advocate combination therapy. Doing effective psychotherapy can be difficult when the patients' brains are numbed by psychoactive substances, which may render them unable to think clearly or to evaluate themselves. As noted earlier, the lack of insight into feelings, thoughts and behaviors is called medication spellbinding.[8,9] The main biasing effect of medication spellbinding is that the patients underestimate the harms of psychiatric drugs.

I shall not go into detail about psychotherapy. There are many competing schools and methods, and it is not so important which method you use. It is far more important that you are a good listener and meet your fellow human being where that person is, as Danish philosopher Søren Kierkegaard advised us to do two centuries ago. As there are many trials with cognitive behavioral therapy, this tends to be the preferred method, but if used too indiscriminately, it can degenerate into a sort of cook-book approach that pays too little attention to the concrete patient's special circumstances, wishes and history.

When we wanted to study the effect of psychotherapy on suicide risk, my oldest daughter and I focused on cognitive behavioral therapy for the simple reason that most of the trials had used this method. As noted earlier, we found that psychotherapy halves the risk of a new suicide attempt in people acutely admitted after a suicide attempt.[10] This is a very important result that is not limited to cognitive behavioral therapy. Emotion regulation psychotherapy and dialectical behavior psychotherapy are also effective for people who harm themselves.[11]

Psychotherapy seems to be useful for the whole range of psychiatric disorders, also psychoses.[1,12] A comparison between Lappland and Stockholm illustrates the difference between an empathic approach and immediately enforcing drugs upon patients with a first-episode psychosis.[13,14] The Open Dialogue Family and Network Approach in Lappland aims at treating psychotic patients in their homes, and the treatment involves the patient's social network and starts within 24 hours after contact.[13] The patients were closely comparable to those in Stockholm, but in Stockholm, 93% were treated with psychosis pills against only 33% in Lappland, and five years later, ongoing use was 75% versus 17%. After five years, 62% in Stockholm versus 19% in Lappland were on disability allowance or sick leave, and the use of hospital beds had also been much higher in Stockholm, 110 versus only 31 days, on average. It was not a randomized comparison, but the results are so strikingly different that it would irresponsible to dismiss them. There are many other results supporting the non-drug approach,[1] and the Open Dialogue model is now gaining momentum in several countries.

Psychotherapy does not work for everyone. We need to accept that some people cannot be helped no matter what we do, which is true also in other areas of healthcare. Some therapists are not so competent or do not work well with some patients; it may therefore be necessary to try more than one therapist.

Like all interventions, psychotherapy can also be harmful. Child soldiers in Uganda who were forced to commit the most horrible atrocities have survived the psychological trauma remarkably well by avoidant coping.[15] If a therapist had insisted on confronting these people with their encapsulated trauma, it could have backfired quite badly. In somatic medicine, a healing wound should most often be left alone, and human beings have a remarkable capacity for self-healing, both physically and psychologically. Obviously, if the healing goes badly, e.g. because a broken bone was not appropriately put together, or a trauma continues preventing the patient from living a full life, it may be necessary to open the wound.

Physical and emotional pain have similarities. Just like we need physical pain in order to avoid dangers, we need emotional pain to guide us in life.[16] Acute conditions like psychoses and depression are often related to trauma and tend to self-heal if we are a little patient. Through the process of healing—whether assisted by psychotherapy or not—we learn something important that can be useful if we get in trouble again. Such experiences can also boost our self-confidence, whereas pills may prevent us from learning anything because they numb our feelings and sometimes also our thoughts. Pills can also provide a false sense of security and deprive the patient of real therapy and other healing human interactions—doctors may think they need not engage themselves as much when a patient is taking drugs.[16]

Being treated humanely is difficult in today's psychiatry. If you panic and go to a psychiatric emergency ward, you will probably be told you need a drug, and if you decline and say you just need rest to collect yourself, you might be told that the ward is not a hotel.[16]

4   Withdrawing from Psychiatric Drugs

As noted above, it took almost 30 years before the psychiatric profession and the authorities admitted that benzodiazepines are highly addictive. Propaganda is highly effective, and the reason it took so long is that it was a big selling point for the drug industry that they were not additive, in contrast to the barbiturates that they replaced, just as it became a big selling point around 1988 that the newer depression pills were not addictive, in contrast to the benzodiazepines they replaced

The lies do not change, for the simple reason that the drug industry doesn't sell drugs but lies about drugs, which is the most important part of their organized criminal activities.[1] The industry is so good at lying that it took about 50 years before the authorities finally admitted that the depression pills are also addictive. Even after this colossal delay, they are not yet ready to call a spade for a spade. They avoid using words like addiction and dependency and talk about withdrawal symptoms instead.

The worst argument I have heard—from several professors of psychiatry—is that the patients are not dependent because they don't crave higher doses. If true, this would be good news for smokers who, after smoking a pack of cigarettes every day for 40 years can stop overnight, without abstinence symptoms.

Patients don't care about the academic wordplays whose only purpose is to allow the drug companies to continue to intoxicate whole populations with mind-altering drugs. The patients know when they are dependent (see Chapter 2); they don't need a psychiatrist's approval that their experience is real, and some say the withdrawal from a depression pill was worse than their depression.[2]

Progress is very slow. In a 2020 BBC program, the mental health charity Mind said it is signposting people to street drug charities to help them withdraw from depression pills because of the lack of available alternatives. Alas, homage is always paid to the wrong ideas people have been brain-washed into believing: "Although they are not addictive, they can lead to dependency issues," a voiceover told the viewers. Haven't we heard enough nonsense by now?

One of the most meaningful things a doctor can do is to help some of the hundreds of millions of people come off the drugs they have become dependent on. It can be very difficult. Many psychiatrists have told me that it is much easier to wean off a heroin addict than to get a patient off a benzodiazepine or a depression pill.

The biggest obstacles to withdrawal are ignorance, false beliefs, fear, pressure from relatives and health professionals, and practical issues like the lack of medicines in appropriately small doses.

Very few doctors know anything about withdrawal and many make horrible mistakes. If they taper at all, they do it far too quickly because the prevailing wisdom is that withdrawal is only a problem with benzodiazepines and because the few guidelines that exist recommend far too quick tapering.

The situation in the UK improved in 2019 (see Chapter 2) but I have seen no substantial improvements yet in other countries and here is an example. In November 2019, the Danish National Board of Health issued a guideline about depression pills to family doctors, which was enclosed in the *Journal of the Danish Medical Association*, ensuring everyone would see it.

The sender was "Rational Pharmacotherapy," but it wasn't rational. As the guidelines are dangerous, I wanted to warn people against them, but I knew from experience that it doesn't work to complain to the authorities, which think they are beyond reproach. I therefore published my criticism in a newspaper.[3] The Board of Health was given the opportunity to respond but declined—another sign of the arrogance at the top of our institutions, as it is a highly important public health issue.

Although the author group for the guideline included a psychiatrist and a clinical pharmacologist, they didn't seem to know what a binding curve for depression pills to receptors looks like. As with other medicines, it is hyperbolic. It is very steep in the beginning when the dose is low, and then flattens out and becomes almost horizontal at the top (see Fig. 4-1 for Cipramil).[4]

Per cent

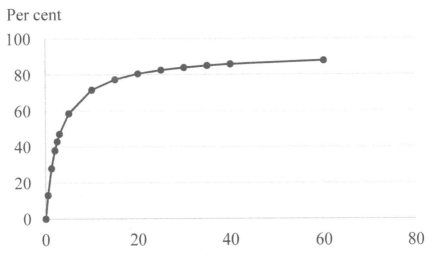

Fig. 4-1: Hyperbolic Relationship Between Receptor Occupancy and Dose of Citalopram in mg
(Courtesy of Mark Horowitz)

This is important to know. The board recommends halving the dose every two weeks, which is far too risky. At usual dosages, most receptors are occupied because we are at the top of the binding curve where it is flat. Since virtually all patients are overdosed, they might remain on the flat part of the binding curve after the first dose reduction and not experience any withdrawal symptoms. It could therefore be okay to halve the dose the first time. .

But already the next time, when going from 50% of the starting dose to 25%, things can go wrong. Should the withdrawal symptoms not occur this time either, they will almost certainly come when you take the next step and come down to 12.5%.

It is also too fast for many patients to change the dose every two weeks. The physical dependence on the pills can be so pronounced that it takes months or years to fully withdraw from the pills.

Fast withdrawal is dangerous. As noted earlier, one of the worst withdrawal symptoms is extreme restlessness (akathisia), which predisposes to suicide, violence, and homicide.

A withdrawal process should respect the shape of the binding curve, and therefore become slower and slower, the lower the dose. These principles have been known for decades and were explained in an instructive paper in *Lancet Psychiatry* on 5 March 2019 by Horowitz and Taylor.[4] Since my colleagues, who have withdrawn many patients, and I have written repeatedly about the principles in national Danish newspapers and elsewhere since 2017, there was no excuse for the people working at the National Board of Health for not knowing about them.

Psychiatric drugs are the holy grail for psychiatrists, and they are the only thing that separate them from psychologists, apart from their qualification as doctors. You would therefore expect huge pushbacks from the psychiatric guild and its allies when you tell people the truth about these drugs and start educating them about how to safely withdraw from them.

This happened to me on many occasions. As noted in Chapter 2, my opening lecture at the inaugural meeting for the Council for Evidence-based Psychiatry in 2014 was immediately attacked by the top of British psychiatry. The Council was established by filmmaker and entrepreneur Luke Montagu who had suffered horribly from withdrawal symptoms for many years after he came off his psychiatric drugs, and he wanted to highlight their harms.

I mentioned Luke's name in 2015 in an article I was invited to write for the *Daily Mail*.[5] It came out two weeks after I had published my psychiatry book where all the evidence was.[6] The editor made many changes to my article and insisted that I added this statement: "As an investigator for the independent Cochrane Collaboration—an international body that assesses medical research—my role is to look forensically at the evidence for treatments."

My research was publicly denigrated by the Cochrane leaders who uploaded a statement that is still up.[7] They claimed that my statements about psychiatric drugs and their use by doctors in the UK could be misconstrued as indicating that I was conducting my work on behalf of Cochrane. They also said that my views on the benefits and harms of psychiatric drugs were not those of the organization.

Cochrane has three mental health groups that have published hundreds of seriously misleading systematic reviews of psychiatric drugs where the authors did not pay enough attention to the flaws in the trials but acted as the mouthpiece of the drug industry.[6]

Cochrane tried to disavow my conclusions about psychiatric drugs, but the organization cannot have any "views" on such issues that carry more weight than those of a researcher who has studied them in detail. But the tactic worked, of course. Five days after they uploaded their statement, *BMJ* (*British Medical Journal*) published a news item,

"Cochrane distances itself from controversial views on psychiatric drugs."[7]

Both then and subsequently, Cochrane's support of the psychiatric guild and the drug industry was widely abused by leading psychiatrists. David Nutt (described in Chapter 2) said during a lecture in New Zealand in February 2018 that I had been kicked out of Cochrane. He was seven months premature.[7]

Luke wrote about his own "career" as a psychiatric patient in the *Daily Mail* article.[5] The symptoms were of such a nature and severity that I at first found it hard to believe him. I had never learned about anything remotely similar to this during my medical studies or later. But I quickly realized that Luke was not kidding and had no psychiatric condition whatsoever but was a lovely person who had unwittingly fallen into the psychiatric drugging trap.

Luke, heir to the Earl of Sandwich, had a sinus operation at age 19 that left him with headaches and a sense of distance from the world. His family physician told him he had a chemical imbalance in his brain. The real problem was probably a reaction to the anesthetic, but Luke was prescribed various depression pills that didn't help.

None of the other doctors and psychiatrists Luke consulted listened when he said it had begun with the operation. They offered him different diagnoses, and all gave him drugs; nine different pills in four years. As it so often happens, Luke reluctantly concluded that there was something wrong with him. He tried to come off the drugs a couple of times but felt so awful that he went back on them. He thought, which is also typical, that he needed the medication although what happened was that he went into withdrawal each time.

In 1995, he was given paroxetine (Seroxat or Paxil) and took it for seven years. When he tried to come off it, he felt dizzy, couldn't sleep and had extreme anxiety. Thinking he was seriously ill, he saw a psychiatrist who gave him four new drugs, including a sleeping pill. He quickly felt better, not realizing he had become "as dependent as a junkie on heroin."

He functioned okay for a few years, but gradually became more and more tired and forgetful. So, in 2009, believing it was due to the drugs, he booked into an addiction clinic. His psychiatrist advised him to come off the sleeping pill right away and within three days he was hit by a tsunami of horrific symptoms—his brain felt like it had been torn in two, there was a high-pitched ringing in his ears, and he couldn't think.

This was horrible malpractice. Rapid withdrawal from long-term use of a sleeping pill is a disaster. The detox was the start of nearly seven years of hell. It was as if parts of his brain had been erased.

Three years later, he very slowly began to recover, but he still had a burning pins and needles sensation throughout his body, loud tinnitus, and a feeling of intense agitation.

When I last met with Luke, in June 2019, he was still suffering from withdrawal symptoms but was able to work full time.

He is determined to try to help others avoid the terrible drugging trap. After setting up the Council, Luke founded the All-Party Parliamentary Group on Prescribed Drug Dependence (APPG), which successfully lobbied the British Government to recognize the issue. He recruited the British Medical Association and the Royal College of Psychiatrists to support this. That led to a ground-breaking review by Public Health England with several key recommendations, including a national 24-hour helpline and withdrawal support services.[8] These recommendations do not only focus on the traditional culprits, opiates and benzodiazepines, but also on depression pills. In December 2019, the APPG and the Council published the 112-page "Guidance for psychological therapists: Enabling conversations with clients taking or withdrawing from prescribed psychiatric drugs."[9] This guide is very detailed and useful, both in relation to the drugs it describes and in terms of the concrete guidance it offers to therapists.

It became more and more difficult to ignore the huge problem with patients who are dependent on depression pills. In 2016, I co-founded the International Institute for Psychiatric Drug Withdrawal (iipdw.org), based in Sweden (now in the UK). We have had several international meetings and have established a network of likeminded people in many countries, and the interest in finally doing something is spreading fast.

I lobbied speakers on health in the Danish Parliament for over ten years and they were always positive when I explained why major changes are needed in psychiatry. But they are afraid of going against the psychiatrists who are quick to tell them that psychiatry is outside their area of expertise. Therefore, nothing substantial has happened.

In December 2016, there was a hearing in Parliament about why withdrawal from psychiatric drugs is so important and how we should do it, which was also the title for my talk. There were contributions from a psychologist and a pharmacist with experience in withdrawing drugs and from a patient relative. There wasn't a single psychiatrist with experience in withdrawal on the program. The only psychiatrist was Bjørn Epdrup who explained when and why psychosis pills are needed—and forgot to tell us when they are not needed—and he said that he could see schizophrenia on a brain scan. This isn't possible. Scanning studies in psychiatry are highly unreliable,[6] but Epdrup left the meeting before anyone could confront him with his claim. The only thing that can be seen on a brain scan is the shrinking of the brain that psychosis pills have caused![6,10,11]

In January 2017, I was invited to give a talk at a meeting about overdiagnosis and overtreatment in psychiatry in Sherbrooke, Canada. The meeting was accredited and counted in the physicians' continued education portfolio. Even though most of audience were psychiatrists, 74 of the 84 participants felt my presentation had responded to their needs. I had not expected this, particularly not after the somewhat tense discussion.

I felt a change was on its way. Two months later, psychologist Allan Holmgren and a political party arranged a conference in Parliament with the theme: "A psychiatry without drugs." Robert Whitaker lectured about the psychiatric drug epidemic and my title was also direct: "The myth about biological psychiatry; the use of psychiatric drugs does far more harm than good."

MIND Denmark Doesn't Want to Help Patients Withdraw

In June 2017, I held a full-day course about psychiatric drug withdrawal in Copenhagen. I had planned it for quite a while, but my initiative was too much for mainstream psychiatry that tried to sabotage it.

The first pushback came when I tried to get an ad for the course in *Mind*, the member journal of the most influential organization for psychiatric patients in Denmark:

"How should you withdraw from psychiatric drugs and avoid the worst withdrawal symptoms? The course is for everyone, both patients, relatives, and health professionals. It consists of lectures and discussions in small groups. Lecturers are professor Peter C. Gøtzsche, child and adolescent psychiatrist Lisbeth Kortegaard, pharmacist Birgit Toft, psychologist Olga Runciman and pharmacist Bertel Rüdinger."

On 6 February, I called *MIND's* journalist, Henrik Harring Jørgensen, who is also responsible for the *MIND* magazine, to ask if they would be interested in telling their members about our course.

When this wasn't the case, I asked if I could place an ad in the magazine. Jørgensen became considerably uncomfortable and said that, being an official, he shouldn't get involved in the debate about psychiatric drugs. I explained that he didn't need to, because whatever one might think about psychiatric drugs, it was a fact that many patients wanted to quit, but couldn't get any help, and this was exactly why we wanted to offer our course, which was for everyone, both patients and doctors.

I did not get any commitment from Jørgensen to get my ad in the magazine. I was convinced that he could not make this decision himself, but needed a green light higher up, and that they probably wouldn't take my ad.

I knew very well that *MIND's* National Chairman, Knud Kristensen, disliked me, which he has told others about, and that he is very fond of psychiatric drugs, which he always praises in the media when I criticize them. When I lectured for *MIND* in Copenhagen in May 2016, Kristensen travelled from the other end of the country to chair the meeting and to ask critical questions after my speech. His questions were unfriendly, and he was very critical of me as a person. But the participants repeatedly challenged him and said that what I had told them was true, for example about withdrawal symptoms and how difficult it is to stop psychiatric drugs, which they had experienced themselves.

I sent my ad to Jørgensen the day after I had talked to him on the phone. Total silence. I called several times and was switched to Jørgensen by the secretary who said he was in his office, but he didn't pick up the phone when it was me calling. I sent a message that he should call, which he didn't do.

I got increasingly nervous because the *MIND* magazine only comes out every two months and the deadline for the ad was 2 March. It was my only opportunity to advertise in the magazine.

On 17 February, I wrote to Jørgensen, noting that he didn't pick up the phone when I called him. I told him that many of *MIND's* members write to me and ask who they should go to for help with psychiatric drug withdrawal. I also wrote to the general email address of the association, but still no reply.

On 22 February, I went to *MIND's* headquarters to get an answer. I met with three people outside who were making documentaries about psychiatry and who joined me into the building.

It became clear immediately that *MIND* did not want to announce our course. *MIND's* director, Ole Riisgaard, treated me incredibly rudely and condescendingly, as when a school master reprimanded a naughty student in the 1950s. Apparently, Riisgaard was also unable to make a decision about my ad without Kristensen's approval; he said he would come back "within a few days."

We all concluded that the director was fully informed about my case before he knew we showed up at our unannounced visit and that *MIND* had planned to prevent my ad from being placed in the *MIND* magazine. When I told him that this was my impression, also when I talked to Jørgensen on the phone two weeks earlier, Jørgensen became highly aggressive and asked if I had recorded the conversation.

The next day, Riisgaard wrote that they would bring my announcement. Riisgaard added that, "In continuation of your very bad and totally unacceptable behavior yesterday where you showed up without agreement or permission, and with cameras turned on filming *MIND's* staff, several of whom are mentally vulnerable and employed under special provisions, the condition for bringing the advertisement is that you, before the deadline, will send me a written (signed) guarantee that none of *MIND's* employees will participate in any kind of broadcast without written consent from each of them."

The cameras were not turned on, and the three of us who were in the room had all been very calm. The only people displaying bad behavior were Riisgaard and Jørgensen, which we recorded with a hidden microphone because it is important to document bullying and other abuses of power.

One of the filmmakers wrote to Riisgaard that his people had followed me for some time and therefore also to *MIND*, and that he had asked for permission to film, which an employee of *MIND* had granted him. As soon as this was rejected on another floor, the film work stopped. The only one who had been filmed was me.

I wrote to Riisgaard that our perception of the events was different. We had complied with all the rules, but as Jørgensen never answered the phone, we had no other option but to visit *MIND's* headquarters to find out if *MIND* would bring our ad:

"You explained that *MIND* is a small association and that you have a lot to do, which was why I had heard nothing. Allow me to point out that there was plenty of time when I called Henrik to inquire about a possible ad. And that it would only have taken him a few seconds to respond OK when I sent him the ad the next day. It is not more difficult than that. It would have been natural for you, when we met, to say that I would of course get the ad in the *MIND* magazine, because it so obviously is a helping hand to the many *MIND* members who want to stop psychiatric drugs but have been unable to get help from their doctor, among other things because very few doctors know how to do it. Other doctors have the misconception that you need to take your drugs for the rest of your life, which is scientifically proven to be very harmful. Instead, you said I would get a response in a few days' time. Do you think this is a good way to treat a customer who pays you to get an ad in your magazine that, on top of this, is very relevant for your members?"

The day before we visited *MIND*, Riisgaard received an email from a local branch explaining that they had discussed at a board meeting a correspondence I had had with Jørgensen about an advertisement for a withdrawal course. "Based on this, it looks as if some form of censorship is being applied. It is our impression that many of our members are interested in Peter Gøtzsche's work. We do not understand this attitude."

Riisgaard replied to the local branch, after we had met with him and had corresponded with him: "With regard to advertisements we certainly have censorship (editing), for example we do not accept advertising from the pharmaceutical industry. But Gøtske [sic] has not been denied the opportunity to advertise. If he gives another impression, it is just to make himself interesting."

Riisgaard lied and continued being arrogant. I wrote to the local branch that someone at the top of *MIND* believes that psychiatric drugs can only be good for people; that no one should get help with stopping; and that the psychiatrists are in control of everything, which they aren't at all.

MIND's National Chairman, Knud Kristensen, has too much power and nurtures his own interests, not those of his members.

The Psychiatric Guild Doesn't Want to Help Patients Withdraw

The second pushback came when I had informed Psychiatry in the Capital Region in January 2017 about our course. I wrote that I collaborated with skilled psychiatrists, psychologists and pharmacists in several countries, and with many users with extensive experience in withdrawal; that we were 11 people from 7 countries who met in

Göteborg in October 2016 and decided to establish the International Institute for Psychiatric Drug Withdrawal; that one of us was a Norwegian psychiatrist who had just opened the first drug-free ward in Norway; that I had a PhD student who studied how to withdraw psychiatric drugs safely; and that we would do our best to meet the needs and interests of the participants.

Three days later, psychiatrist professor Poul Videbech complained to the Patient Safety Authority: "A Peter Gøtzsche, who is a specialist in internal medicine, has announced the course below for patients and others. Of course, it is my view that he takes on a tremendous responsibility, which he has no knowledge at all to bear. Can doctors just do that kind of thing without having the necessary professional knowledge? It is also a private enterprise that abuses the Cochrane Centre's name."

Videbech's arrogance cannot be overlooked. "A Peter Gøtzsche" is a phrase you use about unknown persons, and I was very well known, both by Videbech and by the people at the Authority.

The Authority didn't take Videbech's complaint seriously. It took them four months to ask me for an opinion indicating to which extent individual health professional advice would be provided to the course participants. I informed the Authority on 19 May that there was nothing in the course description about giving individual advice. A withdrawal process takes time, and we obviously didn't intend to start withdrawing participants during the course.

I was also asked about which qualifications or experiences I had with individual withdrawal of psychosis pills. I replied that this was not relevant because the purpose of the course was that we should learn from each other, including hearing about current and past patients' experiences. I added that there would be psychiatrists as well as other health professionals in the room.

Finally, the Authority asked me to state what role the Nordic Cochrane Centre had in organizing the course since I had used this affiliation in my email to the Capital Region. As there was no mention of the Centre in the announcement of the course, I didn't reply to this question, which was irrelevant and beyond the Authority's control tasks.

On 1 June, the Authority asked me for the information I had already sent to them, which they had overlooked. Four days after we had held our course, the Authority announced it did not intend to take any action.

I uploaded videos of our lectures and other information on my homepage, deadlymedicines.dk. We also held several meetings for the public and I gave many lectures, in several countries. We always explained that withdrawal needed to be much slower than official guidelines recommended. Hence, the Patient Safety Authority should have taken an interest in the guidelines, which were unsafe, and not in us!

We considered the pushbacks bumps on the road and in our growing international network, we felt we were moving forward. In October 2017, there was world premiere in Copenhagen on Anahi Testa Pedersen's film, "Diagnosing Psychiatry" (see Chapter 2). She asked me if I had any suggestions for a title, so I suggested that one because the film shows that psychiatry is a sick patient that infects other patients as well. I could have chosen the same title for this book, but I did not want to use the word psychiatry but rather the positive term, mental health.

In November 2017, psychiatrist Jan Vestergaard tried to get a two-hour symposium about benzodiazepines on the program for the annual meeting of the Danish Psychiatric Association four months later. Even though the meeting lasted four days, with parallel sessions, the board declared there wasn't room for the symposium. It was about dependence and withdrawal, and I was scheduled to talk about withdrawal in general, not limited to benzodiazepines.

As the conference hotel is huge, I called to see if there were any free rooms. I booked one and held a two-hour symposium for the psychiatrists in the morning, which we repeated in the afternoon. I gave them the opportunity to learn something about dependence and withdrawal, even though the Psychiatric Association had little interest in the subject.

Then came another bump in the road, which was professor of clinical microbiology, Niels Høiby, elected for a conservative political party in the Capital Region. I wondered why he felt compelled to interfere with our altruistic initiative (we took no entrance fee), as bacteria do not have much to do with psychiatric drug withdrawal. He raised a so-called political question and mentioned that I had written a book on the use of psychiatric drugs and conducted courses to get patients to reduce their use of psychiatric drugs. Høiby asked if the National Hospital's Executive Board and the Capital Region, possibly in collaboration with the Health Council for Psychiatry, had informed the region's psychiatrists, psychiatrists in specialist practice and general practitioners whether they supported or distanced themselves from the activities of the Cochrane Center's director regarding the use of psychiatric drugs.

The answer is as interesting as Høiby's silly and malignant question. Psychiatry in the Capital Region declared that they had informed all their centers about the activities Høiby mentioned; were critical of my offer; and had requested that attention be given to patients that might accept the offer. Moreover, they noted that several department heads and professors had publicly expressed their disagreement with me and my activities, e.g. at the event "The art of discontinuing a drug" organized by the Capital Region and at a public debate about psychiatric drugs organized by Psychiatry in the Capital Region. "At both events, Peter Gøtzsche himself participated."

Oh dear, oh dear, the man "himself" showed up at our precious events and even dared ask questions! So, it is wrong when someone does this and when some eminences—which I call silverbacks as this is how they behave[6]—disagree with him? These are bleak perspectives. Obviously, it is unacceptable for the establishment that I try to meet the needs of the patients when the psychiatrists don't want to, even though the establishment constantly talks about putting the patient at the center of their activities.

I advertised the symposia in the *Journal of the Danish Medical Association* and my PhD student Anders Sørensen also lectured. Later, when we strolled around in the corridors, we learned that the young psychiatrists had been scared away from attending because their bosses would see them as heretics and might retaliate. This bullying behavior is also seen in a pride of lions—if a lion leaves the pack and comes back later, the lion is punished. It explained why most of the 60 participants were nurses, social workers, patients, and relatives. Only seven identified themselves as psychiatrists, but there were likely eight more, as these omitted giving their background despite being asked to do so when they entered the room.

On other occasions, psychologists, social workers, and nurses who wished to attend my lectures or courses have told me similar stories about receiving dire warnings from their superiors that if they showed up, it would not be well received at their department. This is frightening and also diagnostic for a sick specialty. It tells a story of a guild that behaves more like a religious sect than a scientific discipline because in science, we are always keen to listen to new research results and other points of view, which make us all wiser.

We had two lectures in our program: "Why should by far most people who receive psychiatric drugs be withdrawn?" and "How should it be done in practice?" We mentioned in the ad that several psychiatrists had urged us to hold a course on withdrawal of psychiatric drugs at the same time as their annual meeting.

The symposia were successful. The most experienced psychiatrist in the room later told one of his junior colleagues that I dwarfed leading psychiatrists. That is why they didn't want their junior doctors to listen to me. It might become too difficult for themselves when they came back and asked questions. They also appreciated Anders's lecture. He has a lot of experience in withdrawal and is a very good speaker. .

In June 2018, we held an afternoon research seminar in Copenhagen. As guest speakers we had Laura Delano, a psychiatric survivor from USA, who presented risk-reducing taper protocols based on an overview of methods that had yielded the best outcomes in the layperson withdrawal community, and pharmacist Bertel Rüdinger from Copenhagen, also a psychiatric survivor.[6] Psychiatry stole 14 and 10 years, respectively, of their lives and caused both of them to come very close to suicide. Bartel suddenly died in 2021, only 47 years old, from a thrombosis. His psychosis pills had made him obese, and after he came off them, he was unable to lose weight. It is likely that psychiatry killed also him and took 30 years of his life. "You too, Bertel," we concluded.

The Cochrane Collaboration Doesn't Want to Help Patients Withdraw

The biggest roadblock was provided by the Cochrane Collaboration. As noted, my criticism of psychiatric drugs was the direct reason why I was considered by Cochrane's CEO, Mark Wilson, to be in bad standing, as they say in gangster circles, in the organization I co-founded in 1993. I wrote the book *Death of a Whistleblower and Cochrane's Moral Collapse*[7] about Cochrane's recent history and my expulsion from its Governing Board, to which I had been elected with the most votes of all 11 candidates, and from the Cochrane Collaboration. Wilson even got me fired in October 2018 from my job in Copenhagen, which I had held since I established the Nordic Cochrane Centre in 1993.[7]

Cochrane's actions against me were widely condemned and there were articles in *Science*, *Nature*, *Lancet* and *BMJ*.[7] Child and adolescent psychiatrist Sami Timimi reviewed my book,[12] and here is an excerpt:

> This book chronicles how an upside-down world is created when marketing triumphs over science; where the actual target of a years-long campaign of harassment gets labelled the guilty party... Gøtzsche's compelling account includes quotes and documentation from written and oral sources, including transcripts of what was actually said in various meetings. The book stands as a detailed study in how organisations become corrupted unless they have carefully formulated processes that guard against anti-democratic forces taking control, once that organisation has been successful and reached a certain size. This is a book exposing how Cochrane fell into the clutches of a hierarchy more concerned with finances and marketing than the reasons it was created for. The death of its integrity means that the most important institution left that could be trusted when it came to medical science, has disappeared down the same marketisation rabbit hole that captures so much of modern (so-called) medical science. Indeed it was because Professor Gøtzsche was prepared to call out the lowering of scientific standards in Cochrane that the hierarchy felt compelled to plot his demise.
>
> Gøtzsche... created many of the methodological tools used by Cochrane reviews and has never shied away from letting the data speak for itself, however unpopular the findings might be with some doctors, researchers, and in particular with pharmaceutical and other medical device manufacturers. Cochrane under the influence of Gøtzsche, and others like him, became known as a source of credible, reliable, and independent reviews... helping doctors understand what worked and to what degree, but just as importantly what didn't work and what harms treatments may cause. It is these latter issues that meant that Gøtzsche was, and is, an inspiration to those of us who want medical practice to be as objective, free from bias, and safe as possible; but a threat to those who put commercial matters, marketisation, and image as their primary concern.
>
> Gøtzsche's brilliance and his fearless approach earned him many enemies. He is one of Denmark's best-known researchers and is respected in research circles all over the world. But, for years he has documented how many products promoted by

pharmaceutical industry and medical device manufacturers, can cause more harms than benefits; with detailed analysis of how the research from these companies misleads, obfuscates, or sometimes straightforwardly lies in order to protect and promote their products... His work on psychiatric drugs showing how poor they all are at delivering better lives for those who take them, at the same time as causing enormous harms to millions, has earned him the ire of the psychiatric establishment at large, including some Cochrane groups... Instead of congratulating Gøtzsche for ensuring the integrity of the science produced by Cochrane, they began a challenge to this truth seeker for being "off message."

This book carefully recounts this dark period in medical science where a once trusted institution carried out one of the worst show trials ever conducted in academia. The CEO and his collaborators went about their task in a manner that mirrors how the drug industry operates. Its employees are obliged to protect the sales of drugs and therefore cannot criticise the company's research publicly. There are many examples in the book of how once you label someone, their actions can be interpreted as fulfilling that label. For example, after being kept waiting for hours outside a room where a meeting about his potential expulsion is being discussed, an understandably frustrated Professor Gøtzsche, decides to knock on the door and go in to ask if it is OK if he goes back to the hotel rather than carry on waiting. He is reprimanded for entering the meeting and a brief altercation ensues, before Professor Gøtzsche leaves. This then becomes the only actual example of his alleged "bad behaviour" and part of the "evidence" for why he should be dismissed.

After his expulsion from Cochrane, through a majority vote of board members of only 6 against 5, with one abstention, a further four members of the board walked out in protest. Leading medical scientists from all over the world expressed their solidarity with Gøtzsche and outrage at what Cochrane had done. They universally praised Gøtzsche as a tireless advocate for research excellence, a fearless critic of scientific misconduct, and a powerful opponent of the corruption of research by industry interests, and criticised the unsupportable actions of Cochrane. History will recount this as the death of Cochrane rather than the whistleblower.

It was a direct consequence of Cochrane's moral collapse that Anders and I failed when we tried to get a protocol for a Cochrane review on depression pill withdrawal approved.[13] The Cochrane depression group sent us on a two-year mission that was impossible to accomplish, raising their demands along the way to absurd levels with many irrelevant requirements, including demands of inserting marketing messages about the wonders that depression pills can accomplish, according to Cochrane dogma. Cochrane has no interest in a review about safe withdrawal of depression pills but did its utmost to defend the psychiatric guild, its many false beliefs, and the drug industry, forgetting that Cochrane's mission is about helping patients, which is why we founded it in 1993, and the reason why we called it a collaboration.

In 2016, I contacted psychiatrist Rachel Churchill, the coordinating editor of the Cochrane depression group, who showed great interest in my proposal to do a review. I employed Anders, a newly qualified psychologist, but when we submitted a protocol for the review, it was not welcomed. It took nine months before we got any feedback. We responded to the comments and submitted two revised versions, but the demands on our protocol just increased and the editorial delays were so pronounced that we concluded that the editors deliberately obstructed the process to wear us out hoping we would withdraw the review ourselves while the group would not be seen as being unhelpful.

At one point, Churchill attached a 30-page document with 86 item points that no less than four editors and three peer reviewers had contributed to, with individual, named comments. The document took up 12,044 words including our replies to earlier comments, which was seven times longer than our original protocol from 2017. Anders wrote to me that our review was quite simple, as we just wanted to help people wishing to come off their drugs but weren't allowed to do so: "What kind of world is this?"

When Churchill sent the 8th and final peer review to us, her invitation to address the feedback had suddenly metamorphosed into an outright rejection. Cochrane reviews on drugs are about putting people on drugs, not about getting off them again, and the 8th peer review is one of the worst I have ever seen. It is as long as a research article, 1830 words, and provided the Emperor's New Clothes the group needed to get rid of us. In contrast to the other seven reviews, the hangman was anonymous. We asked for the identity of the reviewer, but this was not granted.

We appealed Churchill's rejection, responded to the comments and submitted the final version of our protocol.

Very few changes to the protocol were needed. The 8th reviewer had denied a long array of scientific facts and had used several strawman arguments accusing us of things we had never claimed.

We were accused of "painting a picture" about avoiding using depression pills, which did not represent the scientific consensus, a totally irrelevant and misleading remark for a review about withdrawing these drugs. The reviewer wanted us to, "Start with a statement as to why antidepressants are considered by the scientific community to be beneficial... in treating a broad range of highly disabling and debilitating mental health problems" and accused us of being unscientific because we had not mentioned the beneficial effects. We responded that our review was not an advertisement for the drugs and that it was not relevant to discuss their effect in a review about stopping using them. Furthermore, a Cochrane review should not be a consensus report.

The Cochrane editors had also asked us to write about the benefits and to mention that "some antidepressants may be more effective than others", with reference to a 2018 network meta-analysis in *Lancet* by Andrea Cipriani and colleagues.[14] However, even though there is a Cochrane statistician among its authors, Julian Higgins, editor of the *Cochrane Handbook of Systematic Reviews of Interventions* that describes over 636 pages how do to Cochrane reviews,[15] the review is seriously flawed. I demonstrated this in the article, "Rewarding the companies that cheated the most in antidepressant trials,"[16] and a re-analysis by my colleagues from the Nordic Cochrane Centre showed that the outcome data reported in *Lancet* differed from the clinical study reports in 12 of the 19 trials they examined.[17]

A Cochrane editor asked us to describe how depression pills work and what the differences are between them, and a reviewer wanted us to explain when it was appropriate and inappropriate to use depression pills. However, we were not writing a textbook in clinical pharmacology, we were just trying to help the patients come off their drugs.

We wrote in our protocol that, "Some patients refer to the discredited hypothesis about a chemical imbalance in their brain being the cause of their disorder and therefore also the reason for not daring to stop." The 8th reviewer, who clearly believed in the chemical imbalance nonsense, opined that we dismissed many decades of evidence of neurochemical changes observed in depression and accused us of having suggested with no evidence that prescribers perpetuate untruths to justify drug prescription.

They surely do, but Cochrane used the familiar tactic of blaming the patients for the psychiatrists' wrongdoing and lies. Responding to the same sentence, coordinating editor Sarah Hetrick asked us to write: "People on antidepressants may believe that this is necessary because they have a belief that the difficulties, they are experiencing are due to a chemical imbalance in the brain." The patients didn't invent this lie; the psychiatrists did![6]

The 8th reviewer asked us to explain the concept of ongoing prophylactic depression pill treatment, "a well-accepted clinical strategy," but this was outside the scope of our review. Furthermore, as noted in Chapter 2, all randomized trials comparing maintenance therapy with withdrawal of the drug are flawed because of cold turkey effects in the latter group.

We were wrongly accused of having conflated disease reappearance with withdrawal symptoms, and the reviewer even argued that most people who had taken depression pills for extended periods could stop safely without problems, which is blatantly false.

The reviewer wanted us to remove this sentence: "the patients' condition is best described as drug dependence" referring to the DSM-IV drug dependence criteria. We replied that, according to these criteria, no one who smokes 20 cigarettes every day is dependent on smoking cigarettes.

The level of denial, obfuscation and confusion was really high in the two-year process. We were asked by a reviewer to give references on rates of dependency but had already done this to such an extent that an editor asked us to shorten it.

Our long-held suspicion that Cochrane wasn't interested in helping patients come off their psychiatric drugs had now turned into certainty. But we wouldn't give up and filed three appeals, one to Churchill, one to Chris Eccleston, Senior Editor for the Cochrane Mental Health and Neuroscience Network and a professor of medical psychology, and finally, to Cochrane's Editor-in-Chief, Karla Soares-Weiser, who is a psychiatrist.

We emphasized that the Cochrane Collaboration should not mount ever increasing obstacles along the way for those who volunteer to do the work to help suffering patients but should be forthcoming and helpful. Earlier, we had written to the editors that they "are making something, which is very simple, highly complicated. Our review has a very simple aim: to help patients come off drugs they want to come off." An editor wrote to us that our primary outcome of "complete cessation of antidepressant drug use" should be more clearly defined, as it might not be cessation for life. Perhaps not, but no studies in psychiatry have ever followed all patients till they are all dead.

Our first appeal was not handled by Churchill but by the coordinating editor from the Cochrane Airways group, Rebecca Fortescue. According to her, "a reader can be left in little doubt about the review authors' stance on the relative harms and benefits of psychiatric drugs, which does not fully reflect the current international consensus and could cause alarm among review users who rely on Cochrane's impartiality." We responded with a British understatement: "We are a bit surprised about this comment." Cochrane is not about consensus but about getting the science right, and it is very far from being impartial.[6,7] Furthermore, assessing the harms and benefits of psychiatric drugs was outside the scope of our review. We had not written about this issue in our protocol or offered any "stance."

Even though we had pointed this out repeatedly, Fortescue, the other Cochrane editors and the peer reviewers didn't understand that "Types of participants" were people taking pills who wanted to come off them. As the withdrawal symptoms are similar for any type of patient, disease or drug, this broad approach is the right one, which I explained already in 2000 in *BMJ* in the article: "Why we need a broad perspective on meta-analysis: It may be crucially important for patients."[18] Fortescue requested a clearer description of the population, intervention and comparators, e.g. if we would include trials in migraine prophylaxis, chronic pain or urinary incontinence, and another editor asked for details about which ages, sexes, settings, diagnoses of depression, and types of depression pills we would include, as if we were planning to do a randomized trial. HELP! These demands were totally absurd and amateurish. We included everything!

Although we explained to Eccleston that there was very little that separated us and the Cochrane Common Mental Disorders group after our latest revision, which Fortescue had not seen, he – although being a psychologist – joined the Cochrane ranks and summarily rejected our appeal in just 56 words: "I am very sorry that this title did not succeed because I agree with the importance of the question. I sincerely hope that you will both take what is done and complete it in another outlet.

We need to stimulate a discussion on this important topic and it has become more important over time not less."

Cochrane's Editor-in-Chief, Karla Soares-Weiser, rejected our appeal in 72 words: "I have had a chance to look carefully at the protocol, the editorial and the peer-review comments, together with your replies and the email exchanges between your team and the Review Group editors. The comments obtained from the open peer review process consistently indicated a lack of clarity regarding the review methods proposed and, despite more than one opportunity to address this, the protocol did not show sufficient evidence that this progressed."

We wonder how it can be an "open peer review process" when the hangman was deliberately disguised. We cannot even check if that person had unacceptable conflicts of interest. It was not correct either that there was a lack of clarity about our methods. Even though we found many of the demands unreasonable, we did our best to live up to them, and being an author on about 20 Cochrane reviews and countless other systematic reviews, having defended what might be the first doctoral thesis about meta-analyses in the world in healthcare, and having developed several of the methods Cochrane use, I think I know what I am doing, in contrast to the Cochrane editors.

The fact that patients are organizing themselves in survivor groups and various withdrawal-related initiatives around the world is a clear sign that the psychiatric guild ignores them, which Cochrane also does. Although it is true that "some people get terrible withdrawal symptoms," a reviewer wanted us to trivialize totally this harm by writing that, "some people get withdrawal symptoms that can negatively impact the quality of life of the patient." This must be at the top end of British understatements. We changed "terrible" to "severe," which has been documented using exactly this word.[8]

Cochrane protected psychiatry's guild interests, the drug industry's commercial interests and the specialty's false beliefs also in 2015 when I explained in a *BMJ* paper why long-term use of psychiatric drugs causes more harm than good and that we should therefore use these drugs very sparingly.[19] The same day, Cochrane's then Editor-in-Chief, David Tovey, who is not a psychiatrist but has a background as a family physician, and the three editors in charge of the three Cochrane mental health groups, Rachel Churchill included, attacked my scientific credibility in a rapid response to my article.[7] Several editors of other Cochrane groups told me they were dismayed that these editors had tried to denigrate my research by appealing to authority rather than reason, which they felt shouldn't happen in Cochrane.

We will publish our review of withdrawal in a journal whose editors are not morally corrupt and who have the patients' interests as their first priority. We uploaded all 8 reviews, our comments to them, and our final protocol, as part of the article we published about the affair.[13] This allows independent observers to conclude for themselves whether Cochrane or we are to blame for the fact that the patients did not get the Cochrane review on withdrawal they deserve.

Guide for Drug Withdrawal

Family physicians are the biggest prescribers of psychiatric drugs, but the psychiatrists are supposed to be the experts on how and when to use them, and how to get off them. They are therefore responsible for the drug disaster we have.

The psychiatrists have made hundreds of millions of people dependent on psychiatric drugs and yet have done virtually nothing to find out how to help the patients come off them again. They have carried out tens of thousands of drug trials but only a handful of studies about safe withdrawal. We therefore have very little research-based knowledge about how to withdraw people.

Not only has there been no evidence base for over 150 years on how to come off addictive psychiatric medications—including bromides, opium and barbiturates—but the official guidelines all over the world have been insufficient, misleading and dangerous.[3,9,20,21] In all those years, doctors have ignored when their patients complained of difficulties in coming off their drugs and have been unable to help them.

As a result, patients started to find solutions on their own, and to advise other patients how to stop safely.[21-27] This extensive body of user knowledge, based on the work of those who have experienced withdrawal themselves, is far more reliable, relevant, and useful than the little there is in terms of so-called professional knowledge. I shall therefore focus on user experiences and advice from colleagues who have withdrawn many patients. I will switch between describing withdrawal as seen from the patient's viewpoint and as seen from the therapist's viewpoint.

Many psychiatrists continue to turn their blind eye to the disaster and argue that we need more evidence from randomized trials, but such evidence is unlikely to be helpful, as withdrawal is a highly individual and varying process. Furthermore, isn't over 150 years of waiting enough?

There are many things you need to consider carefully before you start a withdrawal process. If possible, you should find a professional to help you get through it. This could be your doctor, but often it could not. Your doctor is not likely to know how it should be done. Even today, many doctors advise their patients to take the drugs every other day,[2] which will cause horrible and dangerous withdrawal symptoms in many patients and lead to complete failures. Most doctors, and psychiatrists are no exception, expose their patients to a cold turkey because they withdraw the drugs far too quickly, and the failures they cause make many of them decide not to try to help patients again while they convince themselves that their patients are still ill and need the drugs.

It is frightening what happens in "real life," which psychiatrists love to talk about when they try to distance themselves from people like me who mainly get their knowledge from reading and from their own research. But the reality is vastly different from the fantasy world psychiatrists depict in their articles, textbooks and manifestos aimed at influencing politicians and preserving the status quo. Here is a typical story a patient sent me:[1]

> After a traumatic event (shock, crisis and depression), I was prescribed happy pills without adequate information about possible side effects. A year later, I asked the psychiatrist to help me stopping the drug, as I didn't feel it was helpful... When I left the psychiatrist, she had convinced me... that I was undertreated and should have a higher dose... She warned me against stopping the drug, as it could lead to chronic depression. During a time when the psychiatrist had long-term sick leave, I had the courage, supported by a psychologist, to taper off the drug. I had been on the drug for 3.5 years and had become more and more lethargic and indifferent to everything. It was like escaping from a secluded room. Tapering off is not unproblematic, it gives you a lot of abstinence symptoms... When the psychiatrist returned after her illness, she was "insulted" about my decision to stop the drug. However, I was much better, and in reply to my question that I was no longer depressed, she said, "I don't know." "But if I don't want happy pills?" "Well, then I cannot help you!" was the answer ... this

psychiatrist had a close relationship to a manufacturer of happy pills.

It is wrong when psychiatrists' self-respect is related to whether their patients like the drugs they prescribe, and when they see no alternatives to drugs, but it is common for them to dismiss patients who don't want drugs. Although psychiatrists so much want to be seen as real doctors, they have forgotten what it means: *First, do no harm*. With their drugs, they have turned it upside-down: First, do harm. And tell the patients they will get used to it.

It is an uphill battle, but if you are lucky and have a good doctor who is willing to listen and to admit her own uncertainty, you might want to try to educate her as part of your withdrawal process, which would benefit other patients.

Years ago, one of my colleagues, pharmacist Birgit Toft, decided to do just that: educate family physicians. She focused on benzodiazepines and withdrawal from them, and her results were remarkable.[28] Starting in 2005, Birgit made a strong effort towards the family doctors in a Danish region to reduce the overuse of "sleeping/nerve" pills. As recommendations and guidelines had not worked, her efforts were directed towards the doctors' attitude and the renewal of prescriptions.

From 2004 to 2008, the consumption fell by 27%. The model was made nationwide in 2008, and after a few years, consumption across the whole country had dropped significantly.

What worked was the doctors' commitment and change in attitude; that they and their secretaries acquired new knowledge; and the collaboration among practitioners. In addition, it was essential that patients should meet in person in the clinic if the prescriptions were to be renewed and that the doctors' feet were held to the fire by quality consultants in the region.

By far most prescriptions are renewed by telephone to the secretary or over the Internet. The secretary prepares a prescription renewal, which the doctor approves by pushing a button on the computer. This easy renewal of prescriptions is one of the reasons why treatments continue for far too long. The doctor's attention is not great enough when the patient doesn't show up at the clinic. We should therefore require personal attendance for all psychiatric drugs, and attitudinal changes must be made, so that withdrawal becomes at least as important as starting treatment.

Lectures were held for doctors and secretaries, pamphlets were written for doctors, secretaries and patients, and the local weekly press informed citizens that they could expect to see their doctor the next time they called the clinic for a prescription.

The teaching focused on the harms of the medication, especially the withdrawal symptoms. Doctors were urged to start with the easiest patients first, thereby experiencing that it was possible to taper off the medication.

Many doctors were skeptical. However, they had not tried the slow taper Birgit introduced but tapered over a few days or gave the patients a cold turkey. Despite their reluctance, many doctors ended up apologizing to their patients for having hooked them on the drug. Usage statistics were initially perceived as a threat, but when the doctors reviewed their patients' prescriptions, it was an eye opener, and eventually, they asked for the usage statistics to see if their efforts had worked.

Unfortunately, the success was short-lived, as the doctors used the new depression pills instead. Birgit's work tells us that it is useful to engage in the work of practitioners, but also that the effect disappears quickly if it is not a permanent process.

Support Persons

Some doctors will not want you to withdraw. Or don't want to invest the necessary time, as the income from writing prescriptions after a few minutes' consultation is much larger than if they engage in people's withdrawal problems and provide psychological support while they withdraw. There are so many obstacles in the system, which is not geared at all to help people withdraw, that it seems as if life-long medication is tacitly assumed to be a good thing.

Who should be your helper if not a doctor? Try to find a person who has succeeded with withdrawal, a so-called recovery mentor, and involve that person in your withdrawal if you can. There are organisations in most countries with psychiatric survivors that are prepared to help.[22-26] Go on the Internet and find them.

Apart from recovery mentors, the best helpers are people trained in psychotherapy, e.g. psychologists. It can be overwhelming when your emotions, which have been suppressed for so long, come back, and in this phase it can be crucial that you get psychological support from someone who can teach you how to handle the transition from living emotionally numbed to living a full life, so that you don't give up and hide again under a cloud of drugs, forgetting the sun is awaiting you on the other side.

Some psychologists refuse to help patients withdraw because they have been indoctrinated during their university studies by lecturers that are hardcore biological psychiatrists propagating the specialty's many lies. They might therefore believe that psychiatric drugs are so good and necessary that no withdrawal is needed. Most psychologists believe that the psychiatrists know what they are doing. In other cases, they think they are not allowed to interfere with the doctors' prescriptions and orders.

This is not correct. Psychologists may help patients with their problems and give the advice they feel comfortable giving, supporting them as much as they can, no matter what the issue is, and therefore also when the patients have decided they want to come off their drugs. A comprehensive guide for psychologists was published in December 2019 that may help those who are in doubt about what they can do and how to do it.[9]

I know several psychologists who help patients withdraw from all types of drugs, also psychosis pills. Psychiatrists may try to prevent other doctors from doing this (see Videbech's complaint about me above), telling them that, according to the law, only psychiatrists can determine whether a patient should continue with a psychosis pill. What this law means can be discussed and interpreted, but as it only applies to doctors, psychologists and other therapists are free to do what they find appropriate.

A health professional or recovery mentor will rarely be able to support you on a daily basis. You therefore need one or two people who are willing to do this, as you might not be able to assess yourself during withdrawal. You also need to decide whether those who care about you and try to help you can contact your doctor and others, if they observe serious problems or reactions that you cannot see yourself or deny exist. Tell them what you have decided.

The daily support person could be a member of your family or a good friend, provided this person shares your view that a life without drugs is better than one on drugs where you have given the control over your life away to psychiatrists or other doctors.

Your support person should not be one with fluffy ideas, as this might distract you rather than help you. Many well-intentioned people have published weird recommendations on the Internet and in booklets about withdrawal that you should ignore. Drinking plenty of water, homoeopathy, acupuncture, vitamins, other types of alternative medicine, and various diets won't help you.[29] What might be helpful is to focus on something positive, something you like, e.g. playing piano, doing sports or walking in the forest. Avoid negative thoughts as much as you can. They tend to entrap you in a downward spiral.

For the therapist, a structured approach is very useful. There should be ample time at the first meeting, and you should take a complete history in order to understand how you may best help. When did the mental health issue start and what was it? The first symptom is very often anxiety,[30] but this tends to be forgotten, as the condition deteriorates and other symptoms pop up, and especially after a long psychiatric "career" where the patient might not even remember that there was a time when he was well and what it felt like.

Was the patient told that he had a chemical imbalance, that the drugs work like insulin for diabetes, that his disease is in his genes and will last for a lifetime, or that he might become demented or suffer brain damage in other ways if he does not take the drugs? All these lies are harmful because they convince patients they should take drugs they don't like because they think the alternative is worse.

Has the patient tried to withdraw before, did he have any support, or did he only meet resistance? Why did he fail?

An added bonus of devoting enough time at the first meeting could be that you bolster the patient's self-confidence and determination to finally do something. It might be the first time anyone shows an interest in taking the patient's full history, or in listening carefully to the patient when he decided to take his fate in his own hands. This is a crucial and vulnerable moment where you should give the patient all the emotional support you can.

It is often huge work to help a patient get through withdrawal, and it doesn't even end there. You should wrap it all up together with the patient and summarize the withdrawal process, including the most important symptoms experienced along the way. You should also offer your continued support.

Like for most other conditions, withdrawal symptoms waxes and wanes. If you become stressed, some of the withdrawal symptoms might return,[21] which increases the risk dramatically that you will fall back into the drug trap, particularly because most doctors will dismiss the possibility that the withdrawal symptoms can reappear long after a successful withdrawal and will tell you they are disease symptoms. The symptoms can also resurface for no apparent reason or in response to other medications, as many non-psychiatric drugs have effects on the brain. Remember, it can take many years before your brain has fully recuperated.

The patient needs to know that you will always be available for her. This feeling of security and that someone cares can have a strong healing effect (see also Chapter 3 about psychotherapy).

The Research Ethics Committee Killed Our Withdrawal Project

I have had seven PhD students in psychiatry who have produced unique research results of great benefit to patients, but virtually all our results were intensely disliked by the psychiatric leaders and other doctors similarly entrapped in psychiatry's mythology.

There were roadblocks right from the beginning when we wanted to tour the psychiatric landscape. My first PhD student in psychiatry, Margrethe Nielsen from the Danish Consumer Council, showed in her PhD that we had repeated the same mistakes with the newer depression pills that we had made earlier with benzodiazepines, and before them with barbiturates. I have quoted her studies in earlier chapters. They were solid but not welcomed by two of her examiners, who had turfs to defend.[6] One, Steffen Thirstrup, worked for the Danish drug agency, the other, John Sahl Andersen, was a general practitioner.

They wanted to reject her thesis for no good reason, and the third examiner, psychiatrist professor David Healy, disagreed with them. This was a delicate situation, and an official from the university called me to discuss what we should do. We agreed to treat the rejections, which were wholly unconvincing, as if they had been peer reviews. Margrethe responded to the comments and rewrote her thesis a little, and after having appealed to the university, she defended it successfully. If there had not been a third examiner, she might not have obtained her PhD, which would have been a gross injustice, as her thesis is considerably better than many I have seen.

Anders and I decided that he should mentor 30 consecutive patients who turned to us for help with withdrawal, no matter which drugs they took, and write about it because there wasn't a single such paper in the literature. We reasoned that we'd better handle this "heretic" idea—which mainstream psychiatry would be vehemently opposed to—with utmost care and therefore wrote a research protocol we submitted to the research ethics committee.

We considered doing a randomized trial because this is what you usually need to convince people that they should follow your advice when they withdraw people. But we couldn't see what we should randomize to. Short or long intervals between dose reductions? Not relevant, as it is highly individual how fast you can taper. Dose reductions of 10% or 20% at a time? We could have done that and perhaps it would have yielded interesting results. But as we didn't find it likely, we submitted a protocol without randomization that described what we planned to do, for all patients.

Very easy and straightforward we thought, but we ran into a formidable roadblock. The committee responded that, although two experienced psychiatrists were involved with our project, the primary investigator, Anders, was a psychologist and there was no clear description of who was responsible for drug withdrawal, which, for reasons of patient safety, needed to be a psychiatrist.

An interesting remark considering that a member of the committee was a psychiatrist working at the psychiatric hospital in Copenhagen that killed two patients with psychosis pills within a short time interval because the psychiatrists were incompetent.[31] They both suddenly dropped dead on the floor. The first one died right in front of the second one, Luise, who told her mother: "I shall be next." Luise knew the psychiatrists would kill her. She survived for a while because she tolerated the overdosed psychosis pills so badly that she vomited most of them up again. At last, they broke her defense mechanism with a lethal injection of a depot drug. This was called a "natural death." Both she and her mother had warned the department about the far too high dose, but the psychiatrists ignored them.

Every year, on the day they killed her daughter, there is a demonstration in front of the hospital with banners arranged by the organization "Dead in Psychiatry," which her mother, Dorrit Cato Christensen, started. Sometimes, there are around 20 relatives of psychiatric patients killed in the same way.

Dorrit's heartbreaking book about her daughter is one long horror history of wrongdoing in psychiatry. Not even after the death was there any justice. Dorrit complained, but the system's arrogance, both before and after the killing, was unbelievable. She was told that the treatment had lived up to the professional standard in psychiatry, which unfortunately is not too far from the truth, as the standard is horrible everywhere. The foreword, written by previous Prime Minister Poul Nyrup Rasmussen, starts with: "Mom, won't you tell the world how we're treated?"[31] This was the daughter's last request to her mother before she was killed.

So, we could not see at all why, for reasons of patient safety, a psychiatrist needed to be responsible for drug withdrawal in our project. Moreover, it is not a legal requirement.

In order to assess whether the trial was safe for the patients, the committee requested that we conduct a literature review on the risk of suicide attempts and suicide among these patients. This was also an interesting remark considering that the drugs increase the risk of suicide and that there are no drugs that reduce the risk.

We were asked to explain in detail how we ensured that only subjects who tolerate drug withdrawal would be withdrawn in the trial. This was a catch-22 that killed our project, as no one—psychiatrists included—would be able to ensure this. You will have to use trial and error.

The other demands were similarly unreasonable. The committee wanted the inclusion and exclusion criteria to be more specific and asked for an explanation of which endpoints we would use and if our questionnaires were validated and made it possible to draw reliable conclusions. Our endpoint was whether the patient became medicine-free, which does not require validated questionnaires to be reliable.

We were also asked to make a lot of additions to the patient information. Think about it. When a research ethics committee believes it is so dangerous to help patients who want to come off their drugs, then why on earth were the drugs approved in the first place? Aren't they too dangerous to use? I believe this must be the logical conclusion, but healthcare is not about logic; it is about power. .

After the committee had killed our project, I called a lawyer working for the committee and told her that we could just withdraw the patients as planned, without calling it research. She didn't have good arguments against that, so this we did.

Trials are now under way that randomize patients to a cold turkey and to slow tapering. These trials are highly unethical, as half of the patients are harmed unnecessarily. I looked up clinicaltrials.gov for fun and searched on *depression* and *taper*. The very first trial I found was totally unethical, for all the patients. It compares a two-week taper with a one-week taper (ClinicalTrials.gov Identifier: NCT02661828): "As abrupt cessation of anti-depressant medication can cause distressing symptoms (including and not limited to worsened mood, irritability/ agitation, anxiety, dizziness, confusion, and headache), the aim of this study is to compare the tolerance of two tapering regimens with the hypothesis that tapering the antidepressant dose over the course of two weeks will yield less discontinuation symptoms than a one week taper regimen." This trial was sponsored by Emory University, notorious for a huge corruption scandal (see Chapter 2).[6] I need say no more. Psychiatry is a madhouse, but not so much because of the patients.

Tips About Withdrawal

Anders has assembled a consecutive cohort of 30 patients who contacted us for help. We set no limitations on drug type, diagnosis, duration of drug intake, current symptom severity, previous withdrawal attempts, or the treating psychiatrist's assessment of whether discontinuation could be recommended.

About half of the 30 patients had been on drugs for 15 years or more; most of them had tried to withdraw several times without success; and all types of psychiatric drugs were involved. Despite the high odds, Anders has come a long way and has withdrawn most of the patients, in his spare time and without pay.

Anders's work is impressive, and his patients are immensely grateful for his altruistic help. They make *ad hoc* appointments for consultations with him according to their needs, and he arranges group gatherings four times a year where they share their experiences. They have his mobile number and can call him at any time. This is important psychologically and has put an extra burden on him. Many have used this possibility, which illustrates that it is demanding to help people withdraw.

The patients fill out three questionnaires:

1. A qualitative structured interview before the first dose reduction, which includes their history and experience with psychiatry, details on previous withdrawal attempts, their own views on their symptoms and condition, details about what they have been told by their psychiatrists, and fears and hopes for the planned withdrawal attempt.

2. A qualitative interview after having become drug-free about their experiences of going through withdrawal and recovering from psychopathology, suggested guidance for other patients, what the barriers were and what helped them specifically.

3. A questionnaire on quality of life (Q-les-Q) before the first dose reduction and six months after having become drug-free.

Once a year, all patients and their nearest relatives are invited to an information evening where the basics of drug withdrawal and recovery from psychopathology are explained in detail and questions can be asked. The goal is to strengthen the relatives' support function and to avoid having relatives who oppose the patients' choice about withdrawing, which is often an issue.

A peer-support network has been established where patients can share information and support each other outside the official meetings.

The therapy involves helping the patients overcome the difficulties they experience. This includes handling withdrawal symptoms—what they are, how to minimize them, how to deal with them psychologically and how to prevent them from developing into destructive anxiety and failure to withdraw. It also involves coping with anxiety and with the emotions as they come alive again (ceased emotional blunting), the return to society and social relationships, the crisis of realizing how much of one's life biological psychiatry has stolen and using genuine nondrug treatment of the condition if it is still present after successful withdrawal.

Without a systematic approach and support during withdrawal, the outcome is likely to be far less positive than what Anders has obtained. Of 250 adults with serious mental illness who wanted to stop psychiatric drugs, which 71% of them had taken for over nine years, only 54% met their goal of completely discontinuing one or more medications.[32,33] They used various strategies to cope with withdrawal symptoms, which 54% rated as severe. Self-education and contact with friends and with others who had stopped, or reduced, medications were most frequently cited as helpful. Only 45% rated doctors as helpful during withdrawal; 16% began the process against their doctor's advice, and 27% didn't tell their doctor, stopped seeing the doctor, or saw a new doctor. Of the respondents who succeeded, 82% were satisfied with their decision.

In Holland, former patient Peter Groot and psychiatrist professor Jim van Os have taken a remarkable initiative. A Dutch pharmacy produces tapering strips, with smaller and smaller doses of the drug, making it easier to withdraw. Their results are also remarkable: In a group of 895 patients on depression pills, 62% had previously tried to withdraw without success, and 49% of these had experienced severe withdrawal symptoms (7 on a scale 1 to 7).[33] After a median of only 56 days, 71% of the 895 patients had come off their drug. Each strip covers 28 days and patients can use one or more strips to regulate the rate of dose reduction. There is a website dedicated to this where updated information can be found: taperingstrip.org.

Venlafaxine (Effexor) can be a particularly difficult drug, but Groot and van Os showed that 90% of 810 patients who started on the lowest available dose, 37.5 mg, tapered off in three months or less.[21] Some needed more than half a year, as they suffered from severe withdrawal symptoms, and many of those who succeeded in just three months would have benefitted from a longer period of withdrawal, as withdrawal symptoms can be markedly reduced if the taper takes over six months.[34]

However, there is an insurance problem. The Dutch health insurers refuse to reimburse tapering medication for so long because "there is no evidence in the literature" that such slow withdrawal is needed. The Dutch National Healthcare Institute has sided with the health insurers in all cases where patients have issued an official complaint, even when their doctors had attested to the severity of their withdrawal symptoms.[21].

1. WARNING! Psychiatric drugs are addictive. Never stop them abruptly because withdrawal reactions may consist of severe emotional and physical symptoms that can be dangerous and lead to suicide, violence, and homicide.[6]

2. Never try to taper off a patient who doesn't have a genuine wish of becoming drug-free. It won't work.

3. It is of utmost importance that YOU are in charge of the withdrawal. Don't go faster than you can muster.

4. Find someone who can follow you closely during withdrawal, as you might not notice yourself if you become irritable or restless, which are some of the danger signals.

5. Withdrawal could be the worst experience of your life. You therefore need to be ready for it. You shouldn't start if you are overworked or stressed, which could worsen the withdrawal symptoms.

6. Always remember, particularly if it gets rough, that there is a drug-free life on the other side that is better, and which you deserve.

7. It is not your fault if you feel miserable. It is your doctor's fault who prescribed the drugs for you. Don't lose hope or your self-confidence.

8. Don't believe doctors who tell you that you feel miserable because your disease has come back. This is very rarely the case. If the symptoms come quickly and you feel better within hours of increasing the dose again, it is because you have abstinence symptoms, not because your disease has come back.

In 2017, Sørensen, Rüdinger, Toft and I wrote a short guide to psychiatric drug withdrawal, with tips about how to divide tablets and capsules, and made an abstinence chart (see Table 4-1). We updated the information in 2020 on my website, deadlymedicines.dk, where there is also a list of people from several countries who are willing to help people withdraw, and links to videos of our lectures on withdrawal in 2017.[35]

I will expand on this information below. I have been inspired by many people, in addition to numerous patients and the professionals already mentioned, particularly by psychiatrists Jens Frydenlund and Peter Breggin whose book about psychiatric drug withdrawal is very useful.[36]

There is huge overlap in withdrawal symptoms between different drug classes, and although there are important differences, it is easier to follow the guidance if it is the same for all drugs. As it is highly variable what different people experience, even when they withdraw from the same drug, this also speaks for keeping the advice general. You may therefore use my advice if you are on psychosis pills, lithium, sedatives, sleeping pills, depression pills, speed-like drugs or anti-epileptics.

Before starting a withdrawal process, you must prepare very carefully. Make yourself familiar with the type of withdrawal symptoms, in the form of physical symptoms and unexpected feelings and thoughts, you may experience. Read the package insert for your drug and ensure you have good support from persons close to you. You must be determined to come off your drugs, as it might not be easy.

Withdrawal symptoms are positive, as they mean that your body is about to become normal again. They do not mean "me without drugs" but "me on my way out of drugs." During a slow taper, withdrawal symptoms will disappear in most people after a few days or 1-2 weeks.

As already noted, withdrawal symptoms can suddenly reappear after a symptom-free period, e.g. if you become stressed.[36] This is normal and does not mean your disease has come back.

It is important that you get a successful start. It is therefore often best to remove the most recently started drug,[36] as withdrawal gets harder the longer you have been on a drug.[33,36] It is also important to withdraw psychosis pills and lithium early on, as they cause so many harms.[36] Withdrawal can cause sleeping problems, which is a good reason to remove sleep aids last.

It is not advisable to withdraw more than one drug at a time, as it makes it difficult to find out which drug causes the withdrawal symptoms.

It is rarely a good idea to substitute one drug for another, even if the new drug has a longer half-life in the body and would be expected to be easier to work with. Some doctors do this, but a switch can lead to withdrawal problems or the opposite, overdosing, as it is hard to know which doses should be used for the two drugs during the transition phase. But it may be necessary, e.g. if the tablet or capsule cannot be split (see below).

It is generally not advisable to introduce a new drug, e.g. a sleeping pill if the withdrawal symptoms make sleep difficult. If the troubles become unendurable, it is better to increase the dose a little before trying to reduce again, this time by a smaller amount or with longer intervals, or both. You decide, as you are in charge of your drug withdrawal; all others are your helpers.

How slow should you go? As most patients are considerably overdosed, it might be tempting to take a big step the first time and reduce the dose by 50%. But it is better to go slow from the start, not only because it makes you feel you can handle the withdrawal, but also because it can go wrong with a big first step. This could be because all drugs are nonspecific. They have effects on many receptors,[34] and we don't know the binding curves for all these receptors. Perhaps you are already on the steep part of the curve for one of the receptors when you start, or perhaps you are on the steep part in particular regions of the brain.

Withdrawal is NOT an academic exercise that can be derived from theory or randomized trials, it is a trial and error process for every single patient. The pace depends on the drug, in particular on its half-life, which is how long it takes for the serum concentration to be halved. The variation from patient to patient is huge, also genetically, in terms of how quickly they metabolize a drug. Anders found five randomized trials, but they are all problematic. Most importantly, the tapering was too fast in the tapering group, e.g. only two weeks. These trials have led to the erroneous claim that there would be no significant advantage of slow tapering compared to abrupt discontinuation![21]

The dose reduction should follow a hyperbolic curve (see figure 4-2). This sounds complicated but it isn't. It just means that you reduce the dose every time you taper by removing the same percentage of your previous dose. Thus, if you reduce the dose by 20% each time, and you have come down to about 50%, then you should remove 20% again next time, which means that you now come down to 40% of the starting dose. You may need a nail file to do this and a scale so that you can weigh the amounts. Consult the pharmacy about dividing tablets or opening capsules; it sells a tablet divider.

Dose

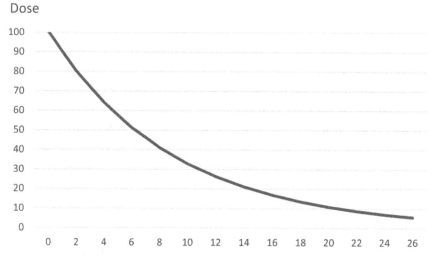

Fig. 4-2: Hyperbolic Curve for Biweekly Dose Reductions

The official recommendations are not like this. They may recommend you halve the dose every time, which means that, starting with 100%, which is your usual dose, you go down to 50%, 25% and 12.5% of your usual dose in just three steps, which is much too fast. Using the percentage method instead, tapering 20% at a time, it will look like this after three steps: 100%, 80%, 64% and 51%.

You can try an interval of two weeks between dose reductions. If it works well, you may decrease this interval, e.g. to ten days. You might also need to go slower than 20%, as you might feel better by only reducing with 10% at a time, or you might need an interval of four weeks.[34]

The layperson withdrawal community has found that the least disruptive taper is when you reduce the dose by only 5-10% per month.[23] However, if you reduce by 10% per month, it will take two years before you come down to 8% of your starting dose, so if you are on four drugs, it may take you eight years to become medicine-free. It is preferable to go faster than this, enduring what comes, and get a new life faster, also because the longer you take a drug, the greater the risk of permanent brain damage, and the harder it is to come off the drug.

Continue at your own speed—according to what you feel. Don't reduce again before you feel stabilized on the previous dose. You may even want to pause on a given dose if you feel stressed. Try to be comfortable with what you do. If the withdrawal symptoms are bad, try to endure them a little longer, knowing that they will usually become less intensive rather quickly. If you endure the symptoms, it might give you an inner strength and belief that you can do it till the end and won't fall back into the drug trap. But if it becomes too hard, go back on the previous dose, and reduce the pace of withdrawal.

Always make sure you have one or two friends or family members with whom you can discuss your withdrawal and who can observe you. You might not notice if you have become irritable or restless, which can be symptoms of danger.

It is not uncommon that people don't notice the progress they are making before very late in the process, and they might tend to focus on the unpleasant withdrawal symptoms. Be patient and endure it. Do something good for yourself. One day, you might suddenly notice the birds are singing, for the first time in years. Then you know you are on the right track towards healing.

The last small step can be the worst, not only because of physical issues but also for psychological reasons. You may ask yourself: "I have taken this pill for so long; dare I take the last small step? Who am I when I don't take the pill?" It doesn't help if your doctor laughs at you and tells you that it's impossible that you can have any withdrawal symptoms when the dose is so low.[37] If your doctor is involved in your withdrawal and behaves like a "know-it-all" guy, then drop your doctor. Having come so far, you are likely to know much more about withdrawal than your doctor.

It is prudent to go down to a very low dose before you stop. Citalopram (Cipramil), for example, is recommended to be used at dosages of 20 or 40 mg daily, and it will surprise any doctor to know that even at a dose as low as 0.4 mg, 10% of the serotonin receptors are still being occupied,[34] which means that you might still experience withdrawal symptoms when you go from that small dose to nothing. Psychiatrist Mark Horowitz admitted that if patients had come to him before he had experienced the withdrawal symptoms himself, he would probably not have believed them when they said they had real trouble coming off a depression pill.[37]

Don't take it as a defeat if you fail; just try again some other time. Tell yourself that you deserve to have a good life and be determined to get it.

List of Withdrawal Symptoms You May Experience

This list isn't complete, and cannot be complete, as there are so many different withdrawal symptoms, but we have assembled the most typical ones. Some people feel withdrawal symptoms very clearly, others hardly notice them. They can be worse than anything you have ever experienced before; they can be completely new symptoms; they can be similar to the condition for which you were treated, which will make most doctors conclude you are still ill and need the drug, even if this is rarely the case; they can be symptoms that will make psychiatrists give you additional diagnoses; and they can be the same for widely different drugs, e.g. mania.

When withdrawing, you and your relatives may be surprised that thoughts, feelings, and actions may change. This is normal but can be unpleasant. You may not realise if you have become emotionally unstable; in fact, it is quite common patients don't notice this.

Below are the most important symptoms you may experience. A few of them can be dangerous, see the warnings in the package insert for the drug you are tapering off. If you haven't spared it, you can find it on the Internet, e.g. *duloxetine fda* or *duloxetine package insert*.

- Flu-like symptoms: Joint and muscle pain, fever, cold sweats, running nose, sore eyes.

- Headache: Headache, migraine, electric shock sensations/ head zaps.

- Balance: Dizziness, imbalance, unsteady walking, "hangover" or a feeling of motion sickness.

- Joints and muscles: Stiffness, numbness or burning feeling, cramps, twitches, tremor, uncontrollable mouth movements.

- Senses: Tingling in the skin, pain, low pain threshold, restless legs, difficulty sitting still, blurred vision, light and sound hypersensitivity, tension around the eyes, ringing in the ears, tinnitus, slurred speech, taste and smell changes, salivation.

- Stomach, gut and appetite: Nausea, vomiting, diarrhea, abdominal pain, bloating, increased or decreased appetite.

- Mood: Mood swings, depression, crying, sense of inadequacy, lack of self-confidence, euphoria or mania.

- Anxiety: Anxiety attacks, panic, agitation, chest pain, shallow breathing, sweating, palpitations. .

- Perception of reality: Feeling of alienation and unreality, being inside a secluded room, visual and auditory hallucinations, delusions, psychosis.

- Irritability and aggression: Irritability, aggression, angry outbursts, impulsiveness, suicidal thoughts, self-harm, thoughts about harming others.

- Memory and confusion: Confusion, poor concentration, loss of memory.

- Sleep: Difficulty falling asleep, insomnia, waking up early, intense dreams, nightmares that are sometimes violent.

- Energy : Low energy, restlessness, hyperactivity.

On the next page, there is an abstinence chart where you may register the withdrawal symptoms you experience and their severity.

Its primary function is not so much to track daily symptoms as to remind you about what the withdrawal symptoms are likely to be, thereby telling you that what you experience is totally normal. You should therefore not worry, ruminate, or panic about these symptoms, but accept them, unless they are dangerous and increase the risk of suicide and violence, in which case a temporary dose increase might be needed. We do not recommend that you do this every day, as it would imply an inner focus and constant checking of yourself. You should try to focus on the outside world, telling yourself that this is where you want to be, instead of being drugged away from it.

There are other problems with daily recordings. You have no reference point when you start. Some patients will rate the withdrawal symptoms from the first couple of dose reductions as maximum severity because it is the first time they experience anything so horrible. Later, if the symptoms get even worse, there is no severity category for that.

It helps some people to write about their thoughts, considerations, and feelings in a diary. What matters is that you feel safe with what you do. You should therefore avoid people and situations that can stress you and avoid taking on tasks that are not strictly necessary.

After withdrawal, you may lack energy for a while and may not feel like yourself. This is normal. Do something you like doing, be good to yourself, and be proud about what you have accomplished. You might need psychotherapy to help you get to the root of what it is or was that trapped you on psychiatric drugs.

Keep an eye on your mood. It can take a long time before you are fully stabilized in your new life without drugs. You might need to learn relaxation techniques if you feel tense.

All psychiatric drugs are addictive and can cause abstinence symptoms when an accustomed dose is reduced. Use the chart each evening to remind yourself and your relatives that the withdrawal state is temporary; it is "me on my way out of drugs," not "me without drugs," which is something completely different and better than being on your way out of drugs. You may write the severity of the symptoms you have each day (1 to 5, where 5 is worst), but do not check yourself too much; the symptoms disappear most quickly if they are allowed to "look after themselves." Note the new dose below the day you reduce it. You may add additional symptoms on the blank lines.

Some of the symptoms can be dangerous; see the package insert.

Table 4-1: Abstinence Chart for Psychiatric Drugs
(Anders Sørensen and Peter C. Gøtzsche, 4 January 2019)

Month: _____ Year :_____
(Write the day of the month in the first line)

Day of the month										
Dose										
Anxiety/ panic										
Depression/ sadness										
Crying										

Mood swings									
Feeling of being inside a secluded room									
Irritability/ aggression/ bursts of anger									
Influenza-like symptoms									
Stomach problems, nausea, lack of appetite									
Lack of energy/ exhaustion									
Insomnia, difficulty falling asleep									
Vivid dreams/ nightmares									
Agitation and restlessness/ cannot sit still									
Dizziness									
Confusion/ difficulty concentrating									
I am not myself									
Suicidal thoughts									
Electric shock sensations/ head zaps									
Headache									
Tinnitus									
Involuntary movements/ restless legs									
Tremor/ shaking									
Muscle stiffness or muscle pain									
Problems with balance									
Sweating									
Palpitations									
Prickling or tingling feeling									
Itching or blushing									
Sticking/ burning sensation									
Smelling or tasting changed									
Light or sound hypersensitivity									
Memory problems									
Sexual disturbances									
Blurred vision									
Mania or hypomania/ euphoria									
Psychosis/ delusions									
Other:									
Other:									
Other									

Dividing Tablets and Capsules

Unfortunately, our drug regulators have allowed drug companies to bring drugs on the market without having to investigate if problems may occur when patients stop using them and to develop solutions if this is the case.[21] Academic psychiatry is also at fault. It has devoted a lot of attention to the short-term efficacy of new drugs and for starting treatment, but virtually none to stopping treatment. It was not psychiatry but the patients who drew attention to the far too limited number of strengths of the drugs. Clinical practice was adapted to what pharmaceutical companies sold and not to what the patients needed.

The patients were right to criticize why the companies did not provide the strengths they so clearly needed, and why medical associations and guideline committees did not ask the drug companies to do this. We don't all use the same shoe size or strength in our glasses, and dogs get dosed according to their weight in contrast to humans.

In this vacuum, we need to be creative. Pharmacists Rüdinger and Toft have prepared some tips about how to take less than the minimum dosage provided by the manufacturers.[35]

> Warning: The box and the package insert will always describe your type of medicine. If it is enteric-coated tablets or capsules, they are manufactured in such a way that the active substance does not come into contact with the stomach acid. Therefore, they must not under any circumstances be split or divided because the stomach acid will then destroy the active ingredient.

You can always consult your pharmacy about whether your drug can be split into smaller units. Here are a few main rules:

Tablets

Most tablets are regular tablets, and the active ingredient is evenly distributed throughout the tablet. If a groove runs across the surface of the tablet, it is easy to split it. This will allow you to get half tablets. Tablets can also be split into four and eight parts, which is often necessary towards the end of the withdrawal period.

Tablets can be cut with a sharp knife, but you can also buy a tablet splitter or a tablet guillotine at the pharmacy.

If you happen to split the tablets into uneven sizes, you can order them according to size, starting with the largest and ending with the smallest bits.

Sustained-Release Tablets

Some tablets are designed to remain in the body for a long time, and they are often manufactured in a way that allows the active ingredient to be distributed throughout the body gradually. These tablets have an addition to their name, for example depot, prolonged-release, and retard. Basically, they cannot be split.

If the sustained-release tablet has a groove, you may break the tablet along it, but do not split the tablet further.

Many drugs are available both as sustained-release and non-sustained-release tablets, and if you need to split a sustained-release tablet, consult your doctor to switch to regular tablets.

Capsules

Capsules are made of gelatin with the purpose of assembling the powder. They can be opened, and the powder can be dissolved in water. The water will be unclear, but ready to drink. It is possible to prepare the water solution in a plastic syringe with ml divisions, and from this solution you can draw the correct amount according to the dose needed.

Use a 10 ml syringe, add powder to the syringe and draw water up to the 10 ml line. Turn the syringe upside down or shake it a few times to dissolve the powder. One ml corresponds to 10%, two ml to 20%, etc. Pour the required contents into a glass and drink it.

Sustained-Release Capsules

Sustained-release capsules contain large particles or mini-tablets intended to be released slowly in the body over a long period of time. In most cases, these capsules can be broken, and the beads can be counted. Part of the content can be sprinkled on yogurt or dissolved in water with a syringe as mentioned above.

Replacing the Drug to Enable Withdrawal

In some cases, withdrawal is not possible with the prescribed drug because the tablet cannot be split, or the capsule content cannot be reduced. You may therefore need to replace your drug with another one with similar effect, available in lower strengths. You will need to consult your doctor.

Some drugs come also in liquid form, which makes it a lot easier to titrate the correct dose.

Forced Treatment:
A Horrible Violation of Human Rights

We must not forget the patients who, even though they desperately want to come off their psychosis pills, are forced to take them, in the worst cases as depot injections to ensure they don't "cheat" by spitting out the tablets when the staff is gone.

I have argued at length,[6] why this horrible violation of human rights must stop. The psychiatrists claim that they cannot practice without coercion, but this isn't true. Examples from several countries have shown that coercion is not needed. According to Italy's Mental Health Law, the danger criterion is not a legal justification for forced treatment; it is a case for the police, just as in Iceland, where no chains, belts or other physical constraints have been used since 1932.[6] Physical restraint is an enormous assault on patients who have experienced sexual abuse, which many patients have, some even while they were locked up.

At Akershus University Hospital in Norway, they don't have a regime for rapid tranquillization and have never needed one.[6] At a psychosis ward in London, they waited on average about two weeks before starting psychosis pill medication on newly admitted people.[6] In the end, most patients chose to take some medication, often in very small doses, so it is very well possible that it was respect, time and shelter that helped them, not the "subtreatment threshold doses." Germany has also shown how it can be done.[38]

With good management and training of staff in de-escalation techniques, it is possible to practice psychiatry without coercion.[39,40]

There must be 24-hour support facilities without any compulsion, so that the hospital is no longer the only place you can go to when you are in acute crisis.[38] For example, there could be refuges with the possibility of accommodation and where the money follows the patient and not the treatment. We also need social and worthy services for people who are on their way back into society after having been in contact with psychiatry.

Psychiatry seems to be the only area in society where the law is systematically being violated all over the world—even Supreme Court and Ombudsman decisions are being ignored.[6,41] We studied 30 consecutive cases from the Psychiatric Appeals Board in Denmark and found that the law had been violated in every single case.[41,42]

All 30 patients were forced to take psychosis pills they didn't want, even though less dangerous alternatives could be used, e.g. benzodiazepines.[43] The psychiatrists had no respect for the patients' views and experiences. In all 21 cases where there was information about the effect of previous drugs, the psychiatrists stated that psychosis pills had had a good effect whereas none of the patients shared this view.[42]

The harms of prior medication played no role either in the psychiatrist's decision making, not even when they were serious, e.g. we suspected or found akathisia or tardive dyskinesia in seven patients, and five patients expressed fear of dying because of the forced treatment. An expert confirmed our suspicion that a patient had developed akathisia on aripiprazole (Abilify) but on the same page, the expert—a high-ranking member of the board of the Danish Psychiatric Association—recommended forced treatment with this drug even though it was stopped because of the akathisia.[42]

The power imbalance was extreme. We had reservations about the psychiatrists' diagnoses of delusions in nine cases. There is an element of catch-22 when a psychiatrist decides on a diagnosis and the patient disagrees. According to the psychiatrist, the disagreement shows that the patient has a lack of insight into the disease, which is a proof of mental illness. The abuse involved psychiatrists using diagnoses or derogatory terms for things they didn't like or didn't understand; the patients felt misunderstood and overlooked; their legal protection was a sham; and the harm done was immense.[42]

The patients or their disease were blamed for virtually everything untoward that happened. The psychiatrists didn't seem to have any interest in trauma, neither previous ones nor those caused by themselves. Withdrawal reactions were not taken seriously—we didn't even see this, or a similar term, being used although many patients suffered from them.

It is a very serious transgression of the law and of professional ethics when psychiatrists exaggerate the patients' symptoms and trivialize the harms of the drugs to maintain coercion, but this often happens, and the patient files can be very misleading or outright wrong.[6,31,42,44] In this way, the psychiatrists can be said to operate a kangaroo court, where they are both investigators and judges and lie in court about the evidence, where after they sentence the patients to a treatment that is deadly for some of them and very harmful for everyone.

When the patients complain about this unfair treatment, which isn't allowed in any other sector of society, it is the same judges (or their friends that won't disagree with them) whose evidence and judgments provide the basis for the verdicts at the two appeal boards, first the Psychiatric Patients' Complaints Board, and next, the Psychiatric Appeals Board. It doesn't matter the slightest bit what the patients say. As they have been declared insane, no one finds it necessary to listen to them. This is a system so abominable that it looks surreal, but this is the reality all over the world.

When anyone proposes to abolish coercion, psychiatrists often mention rare cases, such as severe mania where the patients may be busily spending their entire wealth. But this can be handled without forced hospitalization and treatment. For example, an emergency clause could be introduced that removes the patients' financial decision-making rights at short notice.

Furthermore, a few difficult cases cannot justify that massive harm is inflicted on the patients,[6] which also makes it difficult to recruit good people to psychiatry. No one likes coercion, and it destroys the patient's trust in the staff, which is so important for healing and for the working environment in the department.

In many countries, a person considered insane can be committed to a psychiatric ward involuntarily if the prospect of cure or substantial and significant improvement of the condition would be significantly impaired otherwise. No drugs can accomplish that.

The other lawful reason for forcing drugs on people is if they present an obvious and substantial danger to themselves or others. This is also an invalid argument. Psychiatric drugs *cause* violence[6] and they cannot protect against violence unless the patients are drugged to such an extent that they have become zombies.

Treatment with psychosis pills kill very many patients, also young people (see Chapter 2), and many more become permanently brain damaged.[1,6,36,45] There are videos of children and adults with akathisia and tardive dyskinesia that show how horrible these brain damages can be.[46] It took psychiatry 20 years to recognize tardive dyskinesia as a iatrogenic illness,[45] even though it is one of the worst harms of psychosis pills and affects about 4-5% of the patients per year,[47] which means that most patients in long-term treatment will develop it. In 1984, Poul Leber from the FDA extrapolated the data and indicated that, over a lifetime, all patients might develop tardive dyskinesia.[45] Three years later, the president of the American Psychiatric Association said at an Oprah Winfrey show that tardive dyskinesia was not a serious or frequent problem.[48]

Coercion should be abolished. This is our duty, according to the United Nations Convention on the Rights of Persons with Disabilities, which virtually all countries have ratified.[6] The Psychiatry Act is not necessary, as the Emergency Guardian Act provides the opportunity to intervene when it is imperative, and the science shows that it is not rational or evidence-based to argue that forced treatmen is in the best interests of patients.[6,41,42,49]

If you are not convinced, you should read *The Zyprexa Papers* by lawyer Jim Gottstein. It is a book about illegal, forced drugging that destroyed patients. Psychiatrists, lawyers, and Eli Lilly lied shamelessly, and judges didn't care. Gottstein needed to go to the Supreme Court in Alaska before he got any justice, and he ran a great personal risk by exposing documents that were supposed to be secret.[50]

<table>
<tr><td>**5**</td><td>## Survival Kit for Young
Psychiatrists in a Sick System</td></tr>
</table>

I wrote this book for patients and their relatives to help them avoid becoming trapped by psychiatry and becoming snowed under by psychiatric drugs, thereby wasting years of their lives, or, in the worst case, dying. But what about psychiatry as a medical specialty; can it be saved from itself?

It cannot. Many books, including this one, have documented that the psychiatric leaders have given up rational thinking for the benefits they acquire themselves from supporting a totally sick system. The only hope we have is if the people protest so vigorously that it becomes an unstoppable revolution.

Given the pervasive indoctrination this is unlikely to happen. There will always be too many patients who think psychiatric drugs have been good for them and who will side with the psychiatric guild, and this force, coupled with the obscene wealth and power the drug industry has accumulated by selling useless pills to us, is so great that our politicians, even if they have realized how bad it all is, don't dare act accordingly. The system is locked, as if it had been forced into a straitjacket.

It is also very convenient for politicians that there is a profession that deals with the most disturbing elements in our societies and exert tight social control over them, much tighter than the criminal system allows, sometimes with indefinite sentences, in a closed system where the screams of the victims are not heard, like in the Soviet Gulag system or in the Nazi concentration camps, where the deaths caused by those who held the power were called natural deaths, and where the appeal system was a total sham. What is the difference to psychiatry, that also calls its killings "natural deaths," where the appeal system is a total sham, where the law is being systematically violated, and where independent researchers end up getting fired after a show trial if they try to find out why people died?

But we have another source of hope than the people, the young psychiatrists in training whose brains have not yet been deadlocked into all the false beliefs. Some of them had become so desperate that they contacted me, even though I didn't know them beforehand, to discuss their intense frustrations about a system that so clearly makes matters worse for its patients.

One of them, 46-year-old chief physician Klaus Munkholm from the psychiatric department at my own hospital, had realized, by reading books by Robert Whitaker and myself, that what he had believed in for so many years, was plain wrong. He wrote to me in July 2017 and explained that he was concerned that biological psychiatry had not been helpful for understanding bipolar disorder, which was his main research interest. He had the same concerns about other psychiatric disorders and wanted to do meaningful research.

I am very quick at judging people and immediately arranged a meeting that went very well. We started a fruitful research collaboration, but it had repercussions for Klaus. Already one month after our first meeting, he had—both in an email and at a meeting—been discouraged from collaborating with my research group, and he had been warned that it would have consequences for his career. I responded: "Can you see the similarity to religious fanatism? This is precisely how Jehovah's Witnesses, Scientology, and all the others react. This is unheard of in an academic context but tells us a lot about where psychiatry is."

Klaus didn't budge, and from December 2017, I employed him one day a week, to the great chagrin of his boss, professor Lars Kessing.

The same month, another chief psychiatrist, Kristian Sloth, also unknown to me, asked to have a meeting, and he drew my attention to an announcement from Psychiatry in the Capital Region that depression pills could prevent dementia. They of course cannot do this; research has shown that it is more likely that they *cause* dementia (see Chapter 2). Kristian also noted that he had reduced drug expenses by 35% in just one year since he started working at the department. He told me about a patient who was diagnosed with schizophrenia, received a high dose of Leponex (clozapine), became psychotic, got even more Leponex and ended up in a maximum-security ward. When they stopped Leponex, all her psychotic symptoms disappeared.

Kristian has opened a section in his department that he calls "force-free department" where his patients are guaranteed that no force will be applied to them.

Klaus was a treasure. Bright and kind, a great asset for all the psychiatric projects I had started. It didn't take long before I told him that I wanted to employ him full-time. He finally abandoned psychiatry and became full-time employed, a year after he first contacted me. Some of psychiatry's silverbacks, who had previously held him in high regard, now treated him like Jehovah's Witnesses and Scientology treat defectors.

A psychiatrist quit her job at a department where chief physician Lars Søndergård had overdosed the patients so monstrously, and against the guidelines, that he was no longer allowed to work as a psychiatrist because of his dangerousness.[1] She went to another hospital, but in the meantime, Søndergård had been allowed to practice again, under close supervision, and he showed up at the hospital where she now was.

Søndergård continued to overdose his patients monstrously. His boss, Michael Schmidt, didn't supervise him, and it was pure luck that all his patients survived the huge overdoses, often with several psychosis pills simultaneously. The nurses and his psychiatrist colleagues were very concerned about what they saw and contacted Schmidt about it, but nothing happened. Schmidt replied that, "Many of the patients we meet today in the emergency department are very outgoing and extremely difficult to treat within the current guidelines. It will always be so that the individual physician/ specialist can deviate from guidelines and instructions based on his own experience and the patient's condition."[2] As the culture at the department was one of fear and intimidation, the nurses decided to involve their union.

Søndergård's malpractice included suspending correct treatment instituted by another doctor of alcoholic delirium, which is a very dangerous condition, and prescribing two psychosis pills, which increase markedly the risk of convulsions, sudden cardiac arrhythmias and death.[3] One patient received methadone, which can cause lethal arrhythmias, which is why the National Board of Health recommends against concomitant treatment with psychosis pills, but this patient was prescribed *three* psychosis pills simultaneously, and was dismissed the same day.[3]

Schmidt's reply was extremely arrogant.[4] He could not recognize any of the horrible examples of overdosing the journalist sent to him.

It took four months for the Patient Safety Authority to respond. The verdict was harsh.[5] Schmidt was placed under strict supervision and Søndergård could no longer work as a psychiatrist. Schmidt had approved a proposal from Søndergård that meant that the patients became hugely overdosed, and he had not been able to interpret a scientific article professionally but concluded the opposite of what the article said about dosage. Schmidt had failed to inform the Authority of the excessive doses even though he had a duty to do so, and although the staff had made him aware of it several times. Schmidt had even written to the Authority that Søndergård "has a sharp analytical approach" and had "brought the department to a higher professional level," contrary to the Authority's opinion, which was that Søndergård in several cases had exposed the patients to serious danger.

Deputy Director Søren Bredkjær, the Psychiatry Management in Region Zealand, immediately issued a press release emphasizing that they still had full confidence in Schmidt and that he had only received a "mild decision."

The young psychiatrist in training who had reported Schmidt to the Authority after having tried for months to solve the problems by taking them up with him, Schmidt had labelled "an insane cantankerous person" in front of colleagues.[5]

Eventually she gave up and went to Bredkjær whom she encouraged to examine the relevant patient files. She showed him a list of the patients who were admitted on a day she was on duty and let him see her personal notes. She asked him to investigate the matter, but nothing happened. Then she saw no other option but to go to the press.

To the journalist, Bredkjær beat about the bush all the time and he didn't want to apologize to the nurses and doctors who had constantly warned about the problems but had been ignored, also by himself.

All the young psychiatrists that have come to see me really appreciated working with their patients. I told them they were exactly the type of doctors the patients and psychiatry needed, and that they should not leave psychiatry.

One of them was seriously reprimanded by her boss when she began to slowly withdraw the drugs the patients didn't need any longer, but which he had started in the outpatient facility.

Another wrote to me: "Can you imagine how it is to share coffee and lunch with these people day in and day out, for weeks, months and years? I am forced to listen to the receptor purists' mad ramblings until I cannot stand them anymore and ask them for the scientific references for their claims, and that only makes them angry. I am forced to listen to those that always want to talk about some psychiatrist that annoys them because he is bad at making correct diagnoses until I ask them how they know that their particular brand of diagnostics is the correct one, which makes them angry. Worst of all, I need to listen to the lifestyle-oriented psychiatrists' talks about their apartments, cars, and travels, and they get angry with me if I even mention psychiatry. What I have painfully learned about these people is that most of them are completely uninterested in reading the actual articles about the clinical trials we have. Instead, they simply follow their leader."

As noted in Chapter 2, Danish filmmaker Anahi Testa Pedersen got the diagnosis schizotypy when she became stressed over a difficult divorce. She joked about this diagnosis in her film, and as I had no idea what this odd thing was supposed to be, I looked it up on the Internet and found a test for schizotypal personality disorder.[6] It is defined in various ways in different sources but the test reflects quite well how this thing is described on the Mayo Clinical website,[7] and as they say that the symptoms are published by the American Psychiatric Association's Diagnostic and Statistical Manual of Mental Disorders,[6] I went ahead. There were nine questions, and you should reply true or false, or yes or no, to each one.

1. "Incorrect interpretations of events, such as a feeling that something which is actually harmless or inoffensive has a direct personal meaning." This is a very vague question, and many people interpret events incorrectly, particularly psychiatrists, or take them personally.

2. "Odd beliefs or magical thinking that's inconsistent with cultural norms." That's an interesting one. When a young psychiatrist disagrees with the odd "cultural norms" at the department about preventative treatment of schizotypy, is he then abnormal? And what about Søndergård's monstrous overdoses, which was a "cultural norm," as his boss accepted it? It seems that the normal people in the staff who protested should be considered abnormal according to question 2.

3. "Unusual perceptions, including illusions." I have provided evidence in this book and earlier books that most psychiatrists would need to say yes to this question. Just think about the illusion called the chemical imbalance.

4. "Odd thinking and speech patterns." Surely, most psychiatrists display odd thinking, maintaining the lie about the chemical imbalance and many other lies, and also denying totally what other people see clearly, including their own patients, e.g. that psychiatric drugs do more harm than good.

5. "Suspicious or paranoid thoughts, such as the belief that someone's out to get you." If you are detained in a psychiatric department, such a reaction is totally normal and understandable. The staff surely is out to "get you," namely to treat you forcefully with psychosis pills against your will. When psychiatric leaders use terms about their opponents such as "antipsychiatry" and "conspiracy," can it then be considered a "yes" to question 5?

6. "Flat emotions, appearing aloof and isolated." This is what psychiatric drugs do to people, so if they weren't abnormal to begin with, the psychiatrists will ensure that they become abnormal.

7. "Odd, eccentric or peculiar behavior or appearance." As noted in Chapter 2, one definition of madness is doing the same thing again and again expecting a different result, which is what psychiatrists do all the time. I would call that an odd, eccentric, and peculiar behavior.

8. "Lack of close friends or confidants other than relatives." This is what psychiatric drugs do to people, particularly psychosis pills; they isolate people and can make zombies out of them.

9. "Excessive social anxiety that doesn't diminish with familiarity." If you are detained in a psychiatric department, such a reaction is totally normal and understandable.

There is an amusing spelling error on the website.[6] It says: "Our test will clearly and accurately calculate your points and will give impotent suggestion." I agree that the test is impotent. It is useless and bogus. Many, perhaps even most, psychiatrists would test positive. Perhaps they should try a preventative psychosis pill for their schizotypy?

What is less amusing is that the test provides circular evidence for the patients who, even if they are normal, might test positive when they have been treated inhumanely by psychiatrists, including being forcefully treated with psychosis pills.

A Debate at the Annual Meeting
of Swedish Young Psychiatrists

In November 2016, I lectured in Stockholm and met with Joakim Börjesson, a psychiatrist in training who wanted to do research with me. He was very impressed during his medical studies when a psychiatrist told the students that the psychiatrists knew so much about the brain and the drugs that they could use drugs that were specifically targeted to work on a disorder's biological origin, the so-called chemical imbalance. He found it so fascinating that he decided to become a psychiatrist.

Later, when Joakim worked at this psychiatrist's department, he was asked to produce fake reports that would yield social benefits to his boss' fellow countrymen (he was not from Sweden). Joakim was in a predicament, as this psychiatrist was the one who should approve his stay at the department as part of his education, but he found a way around this where he avoided committing social fraud.

After having read books by Robert Whitaker and me, Joakim realized that he had been totally fooled and considered leaving psychiatry. He didn't and came to see me for three months in Copenhagen where we worked on a systematic review of lithium's effect on suicide and total mortality.[8]

In January 2018, Joakim arranged a session in Göteborg during the annual conference for 150 Swedish psychiatrists in training where I debated with clinical pharmacologist and professor Elias Eriksson.

Our talks were: "SSRIs have a good effect and mild side effects" and "Why SSRIs and similar antidepressants should not be used for depression" in that order. Joakim had invested a lot of diplomacy to have this arranged, both internally and when dealing with Eriksson who has a reputation of attacking his opponents brutally.

There were other issues. During the discussion, I mentioned that Eriksson had entered a secret agreement with Lundbeck (that sells three different SSRIs) against his university's rules, which meant that Lundbeck could prevent publication of his research if they didn't like the results.[9,10] I said this because Eriksson routinely "forgets" to declare his conflicts of interest,[10] but I was immediately stopped by the chair. Later, the Ombudsman criticized the university for covering up the affair.[11] Eriksson stated that he could not deliver correspondence with Lundbeck to a journalist because it had taken place on a Lundbeck server, a highly unusual arrangement, to say the least, and he lied about what the Freedom of Information request had been about.[9,10]

The rules for the debate included that each of us should choose five articles, which would be the only ones we could discuss. Eriksson broke the rules by suddenly asking me about minute details in a meta-analysis I had published that showed that psychotherapy halves the occurrence of suicide attempts.[12] Fortunately, I remembered the details and responded. Eriksson not only broke the rules, but the meta-analysis was also totally irrelevant for the debate, which was about SSRIs. Obviously, Eriksson used dirty tricks in his attempts at convincing the audience that I could not be trusted. Joakim wrote to me three weeks before the meeting that, .

"Elias Eriksson had your book about psychiatry on his article list. When I talked to Elias Eriksson per telephone and asked him why he had put it there (I told him that he could not possibly had found any evidence for the benefit of SSRI in your book) he told me that he had the intention to 'reveal that Peter Gøtzsche is a charlatan' during his lecture. We then discussed this for about an hour and I fruitlessly tried to convince him to adhere to the rules for the debate with no success."

Eriksson claimed in his abstract for the meeting that there was no reason to believe that any of the side effects of the pills were irreversible and that they were not addictive. He opined that criticism of the pills was "ideologically founded" and that their use according to the critics was the result of a worldwide conspiracy that included psychiatrists, researchers, authorities and drug companies. Five months earlier, when I debated with Eriksson on Swedish radio, he said the pills helped dramatically and could prevent suicide in many cases.[15]

After the meeting, a psychiatrist wrote to me that you cannot convince religious people that there is no evidence for God's existence but you can make them lose confidence in their priest if you can show evidence that he has used donations to the church to buy cocaine at a gay bar. He furthermore wrote: "Elias Eriksson is a simple lobbyist that has made a fortune by playing political games rather than doing honest research and he knows this himself. That is why he can lie about things he very well knows is untrue, like that there is good evidence that antidepressants work."

I was also told that many of the psychiatrists had not understood my explanations about depression pills causing suicide. This illustrates the widespread cognitive dissonance among psychiatrists. When I present the same slides for a lay audience, they always understand them. The psychiatrists DON'T WANT to understand what I tell them, as it is too painful for them.

In 2013, when Robert Whitaker was invited to speak at a meeting in Malmö that child psychiatrists had arranged, other psychiatrists intervened and got control of the meeting. They said Bob should only speak about the dopamine supersensitivity theory and not present any data on long-term outcomes. Although this was clearly a setup, Bob went along with it. When he arrived, he was told that Eriksson would be his "opponent," and he spent his time denouncing Bob in an unbelievably dishonest fashion. In Bob's own words: "The whole thing was a disgusting setup that stands out for its complete dishonesty, from start to finish." Eriksson declared that he considered Bob to be a "charlatan who tortures patients."

I had planned on coming, but Eriksson had declared that he would not participate if I showed up!

It is strange how psychiatry's apologists constantly call their opponents charlatans or worse and use strawman arguments all the time. None of us has ever postulated anything about a "conspiracy" or used this word, but by so doing, the apologists associate themselves with a deplorable recent past. Nazi propaganda constantly talked about a non-existing worldwide Jewish conspiracy.

National Boards of Health Are Unresponsive to Suicides in Children

In 2018-19, I alerted Boards of Health in the Nordic countries, New Zealand, Australia and the UK to the fact that two simple interventions, the Danish Board of Health's reminder to family doctors and my constant warnings on radio and TV, and in articles, books and lectures, had caused usage of depression pills to children to be almost halved in Denmark, from 2010 to 2016, whereas it increased in other Nordic countries.[14]

I noted that this was a serious matter because depression pills double the risk of suicide compared to placebo in the randomized trials and because leading professors of psychiatry continue to misinform people telling them that the pills *protect* children against suicide. I therefore urged the boards to act: "The consequence of the collective, professional denial is that both children and adults commit suicide because of the pills they take in the false belief that they will help them."

I got no replies, late replies, or meaningless replies that looked like bullshit to me, which philosopher Harry Frankfurt considers short of lying.[15] After five months, the Finnish Ministry of Social Affairs and Health responded in the typical mumbo jumbo sort of way that civil servants use when they praise a system that clearly doesn't work, but refuses to acknowledge it and to take action: "increased suicidal thoughts have been connected with SSRIs in some studies." This is highly misleading. When all studies are considered together, it is clear that depression pills increase everything, suicidal thoughts, behavior, attempts, and suicides, even in adults (see Chapter 2).

After six months, the Swedish Drug Agency replied. It was all about processes, and I was told that the agency had issued treatment recommendations in 2016. I looked them up.[16] *Under side effects, there was absolutely nothing about suicidality. Not a single word.* Further down in the document, it was mentioned that depression pills increase the risk of suicidality slightly, but we were also told that, "they do not increase the risk of suicide, and there is some evidence that the risk is decreased." This information contrasts with the text in the Swedish package insert for fluoxetine, which mentions that, "Suicide-related behavior (suicide attempt and suicidal thoughts), hostility, mania and nasal bleeding were also reported as common side effects in children." Some of the so-called experts the agency had used, e.g. Håkan Jarbin, had financial ties to manufacturers of depression pills, but none of this was declared in the report..

After six months, in June 2019, the Icelandic Directorate of Health replied that they had asked for an expert opinion, but I did not hear from them again.

In 2020, I wrote to the boards again, this time attaching my paper about their inaction.[14] The Icelandic Directorate of Health replied that they had asked the psychiatrists in charge of child and adolescent psychiatry to give their opinion nine months earlier, but that they had not responded despite a reminder, and had said a few days earlier that they simply did not have the time. I replied: "They should be ashamed of themselves. Children kill themselves because of the pills and they don't have the time to bother about it. What kind of people are they? Why did they ever become psychiatrists? What a tragedy for the children they are supposed to help."

I informed Whitaker about this who replied that he always said that the inaction by the medical profession regarding the prescribing of psychiatric drugs to children and adolescents is a form of child abuse and neglect, and institutional betrayal.

I did not get any replies from Australia or the UK. An undated letter from the Ministry of Health in New Zealand said that the drug regulator had not approved the use of fluoxetine (Prozac) for people less than 18 years of age. However, the lack of approval of depression pills in children is no hindrance for their usage, which increased by 78% between 2008 and 2016,[17] and a UNICEF report from 2017 showed that New Zealand has the highest suicide rate in the world among teenagers between 15 and 19, twice higher than in Sweden and four times higher than in Denmark.[18] When I visited John Crawshaw, Director of Mental Health, Chief Psychiatrist and Chief Advisor to the Minister of Health, in February 2018, I asked him to make it illegal to use these drugs in children to prevent some of the many suicides. He responded that some children were so severely depressed that depression pills should be tried. When I asked what the argument was for driving some of the most depressed children into suicide with pills that didn't work for their depression, Crawshaw became uncomfortable, and the meeting ended soon after.

So-called experts on suicide prevention appear to be highly biased towards drug use and in the way they cherrypick the studies they decide to quote despite calling their review systematic.[19] Suicide prevention strategies always seem to incorporate the use of depression pills,[19] even though they increase suicides, as was also the case in a suicide prevention program for US war veterans.[20]

The title for one of the chapters in my book about organized crime in the drug industry is, "Pushing children into suicide with happy pills."[21] Can it be any worse than this in healthcare, telling children and their parents that the pills are helpful when they don't work and drive some children into suicide?

Censorship in Medical Journals and the Media

It is very difficult to get anything published in a psychiatric journal that the psychiatric guild perceives as threatening for their erroneous ideas. Journal editors are often on drug industry payroll and journal owners often have too close relations to the drug industry, which may threaten to withdraw their support if the journals don't further their marketing efforts. When the *British Medical Journal (BMJ)* in 2004 devoted a whole issue to conflicts of interest and had a cover page showing doctors dressed as pigs gorging at a banquet with drug salespeople as lizards, the drug industry threatened to withdraw advertising, and *Annals of Internal Medicine* lost an estimated US$ 1–1.5 million in advertising revenue after it published a study that was critical of industry advertisements.[21]

When Robert Whitaker gave a talk at the inaugural symposium for my new Institute for Scientific Freedom in 2019, "Scientific censorship in psychiatry," he presented two topics of great importance for public health: "Do antidepressants worsen long-term outcomes?" and "What do we know about post-SSRI sexual dysfunction?"[22] Bob noted that none of 13 and 14 pivotal studies, respectively, about these subjects had been published in the top five psychiatric journals. These five journals did not even appear to have discussed the subjects.

Psychiatry professor Giovanni Fava found it so hopeless to publish results his peers didn't like that he founded his own journal, *Psychotherapy and Psychosomatics*.

The censorship in mainstream media is huge. When my first psychiatry book had been translated into Swedish, I was invited to give a lecture in Stockholm and was interviewed by journalists from two major newspapers. They were highly interested, but as nothing was published, I asked why. Inger Atterstam from *Svenska Dagbladet* didn't reply to my repeated emails, whereas Amina Manzoor from *Dagens Nyheter* replied that her editor thought it would be too dangerous to explain to Swedish citizens that depression pills are dangerous, as they can cause suicide! Fortunately, there was a crack in the never sleeping Swedish censorship, as a third national newspaper, *Aftonbladet*, allowed me to publish an article that filled the whole back page.

When my book about the organized crime industry, which some call the drug industry, although it commits more serious crimes than any other industry,[21,23] was published in Spanish in 2014, I was interviewed by a journalist from the number one newspaper in Barcelona, *La Vanguardia*. The interview was planned to fill the back page, which readers find more attractive than the front page, but was never published, even though the journalist was very enthusiastic about it. I learned later that unhealthy financial relationships existed between the newspaper and the drug industry.

It is also very difficult to get critical documentaries on national TV, and if you succeed, you can be dead sure that the best parts have been removed, "so we don't upset anyone or get too many complaints from the psychiatrists, the drug industry or the Minister." I know that this is the case because I have appeared in many documentaries and have talked with many frustrated filmmakers about this type of censorship. Even after the filmmakers have killed all their darlings so that what is left looks like episode 27 of a harmless British soap opera, there will be a voiceover telling the audience that, "many people are being helped by psychiatric drugs." Really?

It can also be difficult to publish highly relevant books, as the next story illustrates.

Silje Marie Strandberg is a Norwegian girl who was bullied at school from age 12 and was admitted to a psychiatric ward aged 16.[24] She had no clear idea of herself, but the psychiatrists diagnosed her with moderate depression and gave her Prozac (fluoxetine).

They doubled the dose after three weeks. Silje started cutting herself, on her stomach and arms. She became aggressive, heard an inner voice and got suicidal thoughts. She was prescribed Truxal (chlorprothixene), a psychosis pill, and only three days later she saw a man with a black robe and hood who said she was about to die and ordered her to drown herself in a river. She fought and cried when he spoke to her; she said she didn't want to die, but he was there all the time, telling her she didn't deserve to live. She went into the river while crying that she wouldn't do it. She came up again.

She had never had such symptoms until she came on drugs, nor after she stopped taking them.

Psychiatry stole 10 years of Silje's life where it just got worse and worse, with serious self-harm and many suicide attempts. She was put in belts 195 times, was diagnosed with schizoaffective disorder, was secluded, and got electroshocks.

After 7 years in psychiatry, she met a caregiver who saw the girl behind the diagnosis and took care of her. This human effort is why Silje is healthy today.

In 2016, Silje and a filmmaker came to Copenhagen to film me for a documentary about her life. Silje had an agreement with a book publisher about what she perceived was one of psychiatry's success stories. She wanted to ask me some questions, including whether depression is due to a chemical imbalance and what the theory of serotonin was about.

I told Silje that her course was anything but a success story and that she had been seriously harmed by psychiatry. She accepted my explanations, but when her psychiatric "career" was no longer a success story but a scandal, the publisher didn't want to publish her book! The publisher didn't want her to tell that the drugs she was prescribed was the reason she became so ill during her stay at the psychiatric hospital.

Silje was medicated by 95 different doctors. She received 21 different psychiatric drugs: 5 depression pills, 9 psychosis pills, lithium, 2 antiepileptics, and 4 sedatives/hypnotics. This is not evidence-based medicine:

Trade name	Generic name	Type of drug
Fontex	fluoxetine	depression pill
Cipramil	citalopram	depression pill
Effexor	venlafaxine	depression pill
Zoloft	sertraline	depression pill
Tolvon	mianserin	depression pill
Risperdal	risperidone	psychosis pill
Leponex	clozapine	psychosis pill
Largactil	chlorpromazine	psychosis pill
Seroquel	quetiapine	psychosis pill
Zeldox	ziprasidone	psychosis pill
Abilify	aripiprazole	psychosis pill
Zyprexa	olanzapine	psychosis pill
Truxal	chlorprothixene	psychosis pill
Trilafon	perphenazine	psychosis pill
Lithium	lithium	"mood stabiliser"
Tegretol	carbamazepine	antiepileptic
Orfiril	valproate	antiepileptic
Alopam	oxazepam	sedative/hypnotic
Stesolid	diazepam	sedative/hypnotic
Imovane	zopiclone	sedative/hypnotic
Stilnoct	zolpidem	sedative/hypnotic
Vallergan	alimemazine	antihistamine

Table 5-1: Drugs Prescribed to Silje

The documentary is very good, informative and deeply moving.[24] It can be seen gratis. Its title is "The happy pill: She survived 10 years of 'torture' in psychiatry." Silje and the caregiver who saved her from the clutches of psychiatry travel around the world and give lectures in connection with the screening of the film.

Here is another account of censorship, which involved Danish drug manufacturer Lundbeck that sells several depression pills and psychosis pills.[25]

The Copenhagen documentary film festival, CPH:DOC, the largest in the world, showed a very moving Norwegian film, "Cause of death: unknown," in 2017.[26] This is an alternative way of disguising the killings in psychiatry with psychosis pills, the other one being "natural death."

The film had world premiere in Copenhagen. It is about the film-maker's sister who died very young after her psychiatrist had overdosed her with olanzapine (Zyprexa), which turned her into a zombie, as the film clearly shows. Her psychiatrist was so ignorant that he didn't even know that olanzapine can cause sudden death. I appeared in the film and the filmmaker, Anniken Hoel, asked the organizers to put me on the discussion panel. My name was the only one in the announcement: "Medicine or manipulation? Film and debate about the psychiatric drug industry with Peter Gøtzsche."

Seven days before the film was to be screened, I was kicked off the panel under the pretense that the organizers couldn't find a psychiatrist willing to debate with me. It turned out that the Lundbeck Foundation had provided a major grant to the festival. It looks like an independent fund, but it isn't. Its objective is to support Lundbeck's business activities. CPH:DOC never contacted me about it, even though I could have named several psychiatrists willing to debate with me.

The panel included Nikolai Brun, chief of staff, newly employed by the Danish Drug Agency after a long career in the drug industry, and psychiatrist Maj Vinberg who had financial conflicts of interest in relation to? Yes, of course: Lundbeck (and AstraZeneca). She is very positive towards psychiatric drugs and has published utter nonsense about depression being hereditary and observable on brain scans.

Earlier that year, I had responded to statements she had made in a Danish industry-funded throwaway magazine where she had characterized the most thorough meta-analysis of depression pills ever made[27] as "a smear campaign against antidepressants drugs... doubtful populistic discussions... armchair gymnastics... performed by a group of doctors, statisticians, and medical students without special knowledge about psychiatry and depresssive disorders" (which wasn't true). This meta-analysis told us that depresssion pills don't work and are harmful.

I responded to Vinberg's ravings in the same magazine[28] explaining that I had published the article, "The meeting was sponsored by merchants of death,"[29] which included AstraZeneca, one of Vinberg's benefactors.

The panel debate was a total farce. After 25 boring minutes, excepting the filmmaker's contributions, only five minutes remained. A former patient interrupted Brun, who had talked endlessly, by shouting: "Questions!" Many people in the audience had lost loved ones, killed by psychiatric drugs, and they had become increasingly angry because the panelists only discussed amongst themselves and didn't want to involve the audience. There was time for only three questions.

A woman asked why the psychosis pills had not been taken off the market, as they killed people. Brun replied that he wasn't an expert on psychiatric drugs and then embarked on another endless talk, about cancer drugs.

I shouted: "Questions from the audience!" A young man said he had tried to come off his depression pills several times without success and without any help from doctors. Anders later helped him withdraw.

The last question was posed by Danish filmmaker Anahi Testa Pedersen who had made a film about me and her own experiences as a psychiatric patient, which had world premiere in the same cinema seven months later.[30] Anahi asked why I was taken off the panel since I could have made a good contribution. A festival spokesperson replied that they had asked "a lot of people," but that no one wanted to debate with me. Anahi interrupted and named a psychiatrist who would have liked to come. The spokesperson didn't reply but said that since the film was critical, there was no need for me; they needed someone to debate the film's messages.

In the middle of these endless excuses, someone in the audience shouted: "There is no debate!" The spokesperson replied that they would invite me for "tomorrow's debate," which I refused of course, as I had been kicked off from the world premiere of the film.

Seconds before the allotted time ran out, I stood up and shouted (because I doubted I would get the microphone): "I am actually here. I debate with psychiatrists all over the world, yet I am not allowed to do this in my hometown." There was a big laughter and applause, but the audience was angry. It was deeply insulting to them to show a film about a young woman killed by an overdose of Zyprexa without allowing any of those who had lost a family member in the same way to say anything. It was a brutal dismissal and a total prostration for Lundbeck.

Anahi wrote about the affair in a journalist magazine.[31] She pointed out that before I was removed, the organizers had announced that there would be a sharp focus on the overconsumption of psychiatric drugs and on whether drugs were the best treatment of psychiatric disorders. After my removal, the focus was on the relationships between doctors, patients, and industry, which couldn't be a reason for removing me, as this was the subject of my award-winning book from 2013 that has appeared in 16 languages.[21]

CPH:DOC writes on its website: "We have many years of experience with sponsorship agreements that cater to both individual enterprises and to the festival. All collaborations are created in close dialogue with these individual businesses and are based on common visions, challenges and opportunities."[31]

In response to Anahi's article, Vinberg wrote that it was a pity that a debate, which was supposed to be about improving the future treatment of people suffering from a severe mental disorder in the form of schizophrenia, ended in a rather indifferent debate about individuals (me).[31] Her statement didn't agree with her evasive responses during the panel debate

Another instance of censorship involved Danish public TV. Independent documentary filmmaker Janus Bang and his team had followed me around the world for four years, as they wanted me to play a central role in their documentaries about how awful and deadly psychiatry is. Janus ran into a roadblock so huge that he needed to compromise extensively to get anything out on TV. He succeeded to bring three interesting programs in 2019, "The Dilemma of Psychiatry," but the public debate he so much wanted in order to have major reforms introduced was totally absent. There were embarrassing, totally false voiceovers paying lip service to Lundbeck and the psychiatrists (drug exports are our biggest source of income). And me? I wasn't allowed to appear at all.

Journalists have told me that the reason Danish public TV doesn't dare challenge psychiatry or Lundbeck today is due to two programs sent in April 2013.

I was interviewed for the first program, "Denmark on pills," in three parts, where comedian and journalist Anders Stjernholm informed the viewers about depression and ADHD. This was the introduction:[32]

> "In the program on antidepressants… we shall meet Anne who was prescribed happy pills already when she was 15 years old and today lives with massive side effects. And Jimmy at 53, who, after 4 years on happy pills, has lost his sex drive. Now it turns out that he shouldn't have had the pills at all. Jimmy was not depressed but suffered from stress. In the program about ADHD drugs, Anders Stjernholm questions the way in which the diagnosis is made. He meets with the boy Mikkel, who was diagnosed with ADHD by a psychiatrist who had never met him."

The overall message was that happy pills are dangerous and are prescribed too often. But already the next day, the psychiatric empire stroke back. In a magazine for journalists, psychiatry professor Poul Videbech said:[33] "It's a scare campaign that can cost people their lives. I know several examples of suicide after friends and family advised the patient to drop antidepressant medication. Of course, I cannot say for sure that it was because of the media, but as long as the opportunity exists, the media should be very nuanced in their coverage of this topic."

Videbech compared this with journalists making programs advising patients with diabetes to drop their insulin. Even though he, at the same time, fiercely denies that he believes in the lie about the chemical imbalance (see Chapter 2). It looks like cognitive dissonance.

Videbech was angry that he had been left out of the program and complained about it on Facebook and to Danish TV: "It became clear… that they didn't want real information about these problems—something that the viewers could really benefit from—but instead had picked in advance some views they sought to confirm." Videbech described how the journalist repeatedly asked him questions according to his own agenda, which was that "antidepressants do not work;" "if they work, they cause suicide;" and "when you stop them, they cause horrible abstinence symptoms."

Videbech is regarded as a top figure in Danish psychiatry when it comes to depression and he is very often interviewed. This gives him oracle status, which he uses to influence the public agenda and to shape what people think about depression and depression pills. He is not used to being contradicted or bypassed, and this made him angry.

I was the one who documented for Stjernholm that depression pills don't work; that they increase the risk of suicide; and that patients can get horrible withdrawal symptoms when they try to stop them.

There were many commentaries to the article about Videbech in the magazine. One noted that I was right that the media had been uncritical in their coverage of psychiatric drugs. He pointed out that many people had tried to warn against them for many years but had been silenced or fired from their positions from where they could reach the population.

As already noted, this also happened to me which I wrote a book about.[33] It didn't affect me economically since I am well off, in contrast to so many others who have been unjustifiably dismissed when they spoke truth to power. I enjoy my work as a full-time researcher, lecturer, writer and independent consultant, e.g. in lawsuits against psychiatrists or drug companies.

Another commentator found it incredibly manipulative that Videbech claimed that people had committed suicide after stopping their drug and had compared this with diabetics needing insulin: "This is a typical example of the rhetoric that has plagued the debate about depression pills for years... Is it reasonable to harm many people to help the few?"

One noted that it was interesting to see that there were virtually no tapering programs in psychiatry and that it is was solely up to the doctor's opinion what would happen to the patient. She noted that people often end up in lifelong medication.

One mentioned that she was a member of a large and diverse group of people who had warned for years against the uncritical use of drugs and had spent time on helping the victims, either because they had lost a loved one, had seen the life of a person close to them being destroyed, or had tried it on their own bodies. "BUT!! Every time we open a debate on this topic, we are accused of not thinking about those who benefit from the medicines; we are met with the argument that you [Videbech] also use that we do not care about the victims of the good cause and that our information can have fatal consequences!! For heaven's sake, how should we get a nuanced debate out of that???... Almost daily, we are contacted by people, who, also by specialist doctors, are being pressured into taking antidepressants for all kinds of indications. So, something drastic has to happen so that there will be no more victims."

One wondered why we hear nothing from psychiatry about the suicides and suicide attempts that the drugs cause. "Because it gets dismissed as non-occurring. Nevertheless, it was on the list of side effects in the package insert of the medication I received. AND I felt the impulse on my own body. BUT I was told that it was my depression that was the trigger for suicidal thoughts and plans. The strange thing about that was that the impulse came shortly after I started on the drug... But the conclusion from the doctor and others involved was that my dose should be increased, which I luckily declined and decided to taper off the drug on my own. That people change their personality totally—become aggressive and hot-headed, paranoid, etc., is also dismissed."

Only four days later, journalist Poul Erik Heilbuth showed his fabulous 70 minutes documentary, "The dark shadow of the pill," which had already been shown internationally.[35] His research was excellent, and he documented in detail how Eli Lilly, GlaxoSmithKline and Pfizer concealed that their depression pills cause some people to kill themselves or commit murder, or cause completely normal and peaceful people to suddenly start a spree of violent robberies in shops and gas stations they were unable to explain afterwards and were mystified about. The pills changed their personality totally.

About the theory of the chemical imbalance, the background material (no longer available) said: .

> There are very few experts that maintain the theory today. Professor Tim Kendall—the head of the government body that advises all English doctors—calls the theory rubbish and nonsense. Professor Bruno Müller-Oerlinghausen—the leader of the German doctors' Medicines Commission for 10 years— calls the theory insane and an unreasonable simplification. Both professors say the theory has worked as a pure marketing strategy for companies because they could sell people the perception that their depression has something to do with a chemical imbalance—and that taking a pill can help correct that imbalance. Danes who visit the official Danish health website (written by Danish professors of psychiatry) will see the essence of the theory: Antidepressants affect the amount of chemical messengers in the brain and counteract the chemical imbalance found in depression.

Heilbuth had whistleblower Blair Hamrick in his film, a US sales-man from GlaxoSmithKline who said that their catchphrase for paroxetine (Paxil or Seroxat) was that it is the happy, horny and skinny drug. They told doctors that it will make you happier, you will lose weight, it will make you stop smoking, it will make you increase your libido—everybody should be on this drug. Hamrick secretly copied documents, and GlaxoSmithKline got a fine of $3 billion in 2011 for paying kickbacks to doctors and for illegal marketing of several drugs, also to children.[21]

An editorial in one of Denmark's national newspapers, *Politiken*, condemned the documentary in an unusually hostile fashion, and Heil-buth responded.[36] *Politiken* called his documentary "immensely mani-pulative," "sensationalism," "merely seeking to confirm or verify the thesis that the programme had devised as its premise," and they called Müller-Oerlinghausen a "muddled thinker."

The "muddled thinker" gives lectures all over the world, including at a symposium half a year earlier organized by the Danish University Antidepressant Group. He was very clear and well-argued throughout the whole film, and what he said was absolutely correct.

David Healy, the psychiatric professor who has seen more secret documents in drug company archives than anyone else as an expert in lawsuits, was also one of the film's main sources.

Heilbuth told the stories of several people who had killed themselves or others. Already two days after his documentary, I debated with psychiatry professor Lars Kessing on live TV in the *Evening Show* about suicides caused by depression pills. Bits of this appears in Anahi's film.[30] Kessing totally denied the science and the drug agencies' warnings, saying that we know with great certainty that SSRIs protect against suicide. He added that the risk of suicide is large when people stop SSRIs but failed to mention that this is because of the pills' harmful effects, as the patients get a cold turkey.

Three days later, I was in a TV debate again with Kessing, this time about how we could reduce the consumption of depression pills. Kessing claimed that they are not dangerous. Lundbeck's director of research, Anders Gersel Pedersen, was also in the studio and said that the most dangerous thing is not to treat the patients, and he claimed that the patients don't become addicted but get a relapse of the disease when they stop taking the pills. Kessing claimed that perhaps only 10% of those who visit their family doctor are not helped by the medicine, quite a remark about drugs that don't work and where flawed trials have shown not a 90% but only a 10% effect. When Kessing was asked by the interviewer how the consumption of pills could be reduced—no matter what he might think about its size—he didn't answer the question. He said we knew for sure that there had been a rising incidence of moderate to severe depression over the past 50 years. I replied that we could not tell because the criteria for diagnosing depression had been lowered all the time during this period.

I have experienced that when journalists react violently and go directly against the scientific evidence and the authorities' warnings, it is virtually always because they think the pills have helped them or someone close to them, or because a relative works for Lundbeck or is a psychiatrist. I have been exposed to many such vitriolic attacks. It is sad that journalists throw everything overboard they learned at journalism school and explode in a cascade of rage and *ad hominem* attacks, but that can happen if you tell the truth about depression pills. You are attacking a religion.

As an example, a journalist triumphed in her headline: "I take happy pills, otherwise I would be dead!"[37] She called me a life-threatening person, delusional, not in complete balance with myself but a person who might need to see a psychiatrist, and who should be ashamed of myself and be deprived of my professor title. "My wish is that someone can stop the mad professor." She wrote this in a tabloid newspaper, but they shouldn't publish such ravings.

In a radio debate, *MIND's* National Chairman, Knud Kristensen, argued that some of their patients had said that depression pills had saved their life. I responded that it was an unfair argument because all those the pills had killed couldn't raise from their graves and say the pills killed them.

I shall finish with the worst part. I had never before seen an institution willingly admitting that it educates journalists to write flawed articles, uncritically repeating the strongly misleading narratives created by the drug industry and corrupt psychiatrists to the great harm of our patients and societies.[21,38] But there it was, in 2020, in a country that already traded abundantly in fake news.

The Carter Center's Guide for Mental Health Journalism is the first of its kind in the USA.[39] Reporters are told to write that behavioral health conditions are common and that research into the causes of and treatments for these conditions has led to important discoveries over the past decade. They should inform the public that prevention and intervention efforts are effective and helpful. This means drugs, of course, and it is the same message that the American Psychiatric Association has been promoting for over 40 years.

All of this is plain wrong. But it continues:

Journalists should pin down exactly what a professional says is wrong with a patient and use that information to characterize a person's mental state. There is no encouragement for journalists to consider how people so diagnosed *see themselves,* or whether they accept their diagnostic label, or if the professional might be wrong.

Some of the so-called facts journalists are urged to include are: "Substance use disorders are diseases of the brain." The guide explains that, "Although science has not found a specific cause for many mental health conditions, a complex interplay of genetic, neurobiological, behavioral, and environmental factors often contribute to these conditions."

Reporters are not encouraged to explore why it is that the public health burden of mental disorders has grown dramatically in the past 35 years, at the same time as the use of psychiatric drugs has exploded.[40]

According to the Carter Center, the DSM-5 is a reliable guide for making diagnoses. There is no mention of the fact that the diagnoses are totally arbitrary constructs created by consensus among a small group of psychiatrists, or that they lack validity, or that psychiatrists disagree wildly when asked to examine the same patients, or that most healthy people would get one or more diagnoses if tested.

The guide prompts reporters to echo the message from the American Psychiatric Association that psychiatric conditions are often undiagnosed and undertreated, and that psychiatric treatment is effective. "Psychiatric treatment" is a euphemism for drugs, but it avoids any discussion about how ineffective and harmful they are and makes everyone take the bait because "treatment" pretends to cover also psychotherapy, even though this is rarely offered.

The guide states that between 70% and 90% of people with a mental health condition experience a significant reduction in symptoms and improvement in quality of life after receiving treatment. The source of this horrendously false information is the National Alliance on Mental Illness (NAMI), a heavily corrupted patient organisation.[38] It is true that most people improve but that would also have happened without any treatment at all. The Carter Center seems to have "forgotten" why we do placebo-controlled trials, and, as I have explained in Chapter 2, psychiatric pills do not improve quality of life; they worsen it.

Reporters are told to emphasize the positive and avoid focusing on the failures of psychiatric care. The guide does not provide any resources for obtaining the perspectives of people with lived experience, most of whom would speak critically of the conventional wisdom. Furthermore, there are no discernible "services users" or survivor groups on the Center's two key advisory boards.

Unfortunately, the Carter Center is seen as a leader in training journalists on how to report on mental health. It encourages journalists to act as stenographers who repeat conventional dogma.

It is difficult to see much hope for America. The Carter Center was founded by former First Lady, Rosalynn Carter.

No Hope for Psychiatry: Suggestions for a New System

I have explained in this book how I have tried to reform psychiatry, what kind of roadblocks I and others ran into, and what it cost me personally.

I have also tried to change psychiatry from inside the tent. In December 2017, I applied for membership in the Danish Psychiatric Association, which shouldn't have been a problem, according to their own rules: "The aim of the Association is to further Danish psychiatry. In particular, it is a task of the Association to further Danish psychiatric research, to ensure the best possible education of psychiatrists, to work for providing optimal psychiatric treatment for the population, and to propagate knowledge about psychiatry."

I explained that I had contributed to the aims of the Association throughout many years without being a member and that a membership would give me better opportunities to contribute.

Total silence. I sent a reminder after one month, and when the silence continued, I wrote to the entire board, seven weeks after my first e-mail.

The next day, the chair, Torsten Bjørn Jacobsen's only comment in his rejection letter was that I did not work to further the aim of the Association.

Two days later, I sent a detailed letter, noting that they violated their own rules. I noted that I would like to participate in the next annual meeting, which I could only do if I was a member. I detailed the many ways in which, to an unusual degree, I had contributed to the aim of the Association. I also mentioned that during the last annual meeting of the Association, an honorable member held a speech in which he underlined that the psychiatrists needed to communicate with me. The many awards psychiatric patients and colleagues had given me should perhaps also have influenced the board, but they didn't.

Three weeks later, Jacobsen replied that, "The board has emphasized the content and nature of the authoring business you have had over the years, which contains opinions and views on the psychiatric specialty which is in no harmony with the Association's aims. The Association is, of course, responsive to different attitudes within the specialty, though a basic element of a membership of the Association must be that you respect the specialty and accepted forms of treatment, which your authoring business does not live up to."

It is sometimes worthwhile to try to obtain the impossible because it can reveal what people truly stand for, behind the official window dressing. It's like touching a spider's net to see it comes rushing out of its hide in the bottom and reveals itself. This was a clear demonstration of censorship and Berufsverbot. It was exactly what many psychiatrists in training had talked to me about; their deep frustrations that if they were critical of overdosing the patients or the way psychiatrists made diagnoses, they would come in bad standing. The rejection looked like an echo of one of the criteria for making a diagnosis of schizotypy: "Odd beliefs or magical thinking that's inconsistent with cultural norms." Other views than mainstream ones were inconsistent with the cultural norms in the Danish Psychiatric Association.

During the Association's general assembly three months later, Kristian Sloth asked why I could not become a member. He got no meaningful reply, but the audience applauded. I had sneaked in, in the back of the room, and heard it all.

Three months later, when the Association had a new chair, I applied again. To my point that no satisfactory explanation was given at the general assembly as to why I had been denied membership, Gitte Ahle replied that, "We do not share this view because people were satisfied with the oral statement as to why you had been rejected."

I totally understand the frustrations psychiatric patients have. They are constantly being told that what they have themselves observed, is not correct because their psychiatrists do not share their views. It is no wonder that a general assembly that mainly consists of people wanting to preserve the status quo applause a "no comment explanation" of why I could not become a member.

There are many excellent psychiatrists, but they are very few in number compared to the poor ones and they cannot change a sick system. In early 2020, a young psychiatrist in training called for help on an e-mail list for critical psychiatrists. He worked at a hospital in London where biological psychiatry was the big thing, as everywhere else, but he had also met with critically minded people. He was advised that there are critical psychiatrists everywhere. One of those who replied noted that he had also seriously considered dropping out of psychiatric training, but a wise friend told him to play the game, get his official credentials, and then de-school himself. This had worked well and had given him the authority he needed to throw stones at the establishment.

When I published my ten myths about psychiatry, which are harmful for people, in a newspaper in January 2014, I ended my article this way:[41]

> "Psychotropic drugs can be useful sometimes for some patients, particularly in short-term use, in acute situations. But after my studies in this area, I have arrived at a very uncomfortable conclusion: Our citizens would be far better off if we removed all the psychotropic drugs from the market, as doctors are unable to handle them. It is inescapable that their availability causes more harm than good. The doctors cannot handle the paradox that drugs that can be useful in short-term treatment are very harmful when used for years and create those diseases they were meant to alleviate and even worse diseases. In the coming years, psychiatry should therefore do everything it can to treat as little as possible, in as short time as possible, or not at all, with psychotropic drugs."

I got the whole Danish establishment on my back when I published this article, and the Minister of Health threatened that I could get fired.[38] The only thing I had done was to tell people the truth. This cannot be tolerated when the subject is psychiatry, which could not survive in its present form if we collectively faced the lies and acted accordingly.

Outside the power circles, my paper was much appreciated.[42] Numerous articles followed, some written by psychiatrists who agreed with me. For more than a month, there wasn't a single day without discussion of these issues on radio, TV or in newspapers, and there were also debates at psychiatric departments. People in Norway and Sweden thanked me for having started a discussion that was impossible to have in their country, and I received hundreds of emails from patients that confirmed with their own stories that what I had written in my article was true.

Nothing changed. Perhaps a little here and there, but nothing material.

Patient Stories

Here are some stories young psychiatrists and patients have sent to me.

An 18-year-old student was still grieving after his father hanged himself five years earlier. After he was put on sertraline (Zoloft), he tried to hang himself and was admitted to a psychiatric hospital. The admitting psychiatrist increased the dose of sertraline. When a young psychiatrist noted that depression pills increase the risk of suicide, the consultant replied that they were aware of this but had to treat depression, and if the young man committed suicide without being on a depression pill, they would be questioned why he was not treated.

A middle-aged man with symptoms of pneumonia and a low mood was put on penicillin, sertraline and a sedative by his family physician. When the patient started sweating profusely and developed psychosis with mania, he was admitted to a psychiatric hospital, with a fever. The admitting consultant opined he had polymorphic schizophrenia, stopped sertraline, and started olanzapine (Zyprexa) and another sedative. When discharged, the diagnosis was dissociative trance disorder. When a young psychiatrist asked if the psychosis could have been caused by sertraline, he was told: "I've never seen anybody with antidepressant-induced psychosis." This lack of logic kills patients. If people who come home from Africa with a fever are not examined for malaria because the admitting physician has never seen anyone with malaria, some will die. I was in that situation as a young man after an expedition in Kenya.[25] Although I was very ill, with typical malaria symptoms, two attending doctors who visited me in my apartment on different days didn't find it necessary to examine my blood for malaria. I lived alone and was lucky that I survived without getting the treatment I needed.

Hundreds of people have sent me the most extraordinary stories from their life. Some have thanked me for saving their life or their spouse's, son's or daughter's life, e.g.: "It was your book (*Deadly*

Psychiatry and Organised Denial) that gave us the courage to withdraw our son from antipsychotics four years ago, less than five months after he started." I later met with this father who is now very active in the withdrawal community in Israel.

Another patient who thanked me for having saved her life wrote that if she had not read my books and learned that there is something called withdrawal, she would have thought she had become insane. After ten years on duloxetine (Cymbalta), she went through a three-year withdrawal that was very tough and difficult.

A patient wrote: I have used depression pills for five years because of social anxiety. They made my life a mess. Things are now way worse at every level of my life. The pills have changed my personality into being angry and disrespectful. I am more "brave," but it is not me. I would never have started on them if I had known what would happen; I have also lost many friends. Thank you for your book; I am very happy that someone says how things are. The world is so insane. I have lost my trust in psychiatry, drug companies and doctors. I just wanted you to know that people are becoming more aware of this madness. In our SSRI withdrawing group, the number of members increases all the time.

A family doctor used depression pills as a diagnostic test: If they worked, you had depression, and if not, you did not have depression. Another family doctor responded to a question about how to stop a depression pill: "You can just stop!"

A patient was told by her psychiatrist that depression pills were like putting a plaster cast on a broken leg. She tried to withdraw twice in vain and was told she had a chemical imbalance and needed the drug for the rest of her life, and her psychiatrist even increased the dose. A substitute for her family doctor saved her. He said that the pills were devilry and made her sick, and he helped her withdraw. She now wants to help others because she works as a job consultant with unemployed people, many of whom get hooked on the pills because of stress and anxiety.

A father was denied custody of his children because he refused to take psychiatric drugs. Numerous other people have written to me about how badly they were treated by psychiatry, sometimes with derogatory comments in the patient's file about their personality when they tried to avoid that their child was treated with psychosis pills.

One patient wrote to me that a test showed she had an IQ of 70 while she was doped.

Another wrote that her psychiatrist had told her she had an incurable genetic disease and needed psychosis pills for the rest of her life. When she had withdrawn the drugs, her psychiatrist told her she would have a new psychotic episode again. When she had complained that she could no longer concentrate, slept a lot and believed the drugs affected her memory so it was hard to study, the reply was that the problem wasn't the drugs but that she lost neurons due to psychosis and that her brain wasn't the same anymore. So, she needed to take psychosis pills indefinitely to protect her brain from losing more neurons; otherwise she would become demented. When the patient said she did not want to take the drugs for the rest of her life, the psychiatrist replied that she would then not see her anymore because she only worked with patients who wanted to be treated. "Ziprasidone [Geodon] withdrawal was hell. I was vomiting and couldn't sleep for several nights until my body adjusted. I told my father I had stopped, and he wanted to force me to go back on medication and threatened to send me to a mental hospital if I didn't follow the doctor's instructions. He asked me: Do you want to be tied up in a madhouse? So, I lied to him saying that I went back on the medications. Anyway, I am fine now, the people I live with agree and support my decision and the new therapist accepts it too. Thanks for reading a bit of my story."

Another patient wrote: "The psychoanalyst said I had to trust the doctor and the doctor said I had to be on medicines for the rest of my life, but I discontinued all medicines for about 8 weeks, and I couldn't feel better. I am no longer a zombie, I am back to listening to music, laughing, singing in the shower, feeling life, and having sexual pleasure. I am back to being myself. I told the doctor that medicines were giving me anorgasmia and she asked with these words: 'Which do you prefer, not having orgasms or going mad?' That was when I realized something was wrong, as I do not wish to live chemically castrated as if I am going through a lifetime with a lobotomy." This patient had been sexually abused as a child.

A patient wrote that he took fluoxetine (Prozac) for ten years, which changed his personality, and he lost almost all his friends. He went through a horrible withdrawal without help where he couldn't even get out of bed. His doctor told him that psychiatric drugs were vital for him, like insulin for a patient with diabetes, and he started on a drug again, but tolerated it badly. Then, his psychiatrist said that his side effects were likely caused by his depression, and he wanted him to try another drug. This patient had attended one of my lectures in

Stockholm and therefore knew I had a list of people who could help him withdraw, which is why he wrote to me.

Here is my last patient story, told by himself and his mother. It summarises tragically what is wrong with psychiatry.

David Stofkooper, a young Dutchman, ended his life in January 2020, only 23 years old. He had a flourishing social life, was a lively, very intelligent student, with a lot of friends, enjoyed socializing and loved listening to music. Since he was 17, he could ruminate a lot, with repetitive thoughts; not constantly, and he still had a fun life. But he made a fatal mistake. He consulted a psychiatrist and was put on sertraline (Zoloft), in October 2017. Within two weeks, he became suicidal. The psychiatrist increased the dose, and it got worse. He became zombified, with no libido and no emotions; his whole personality had disappeared.

His mother called his psychiatrist and said this definitely didn't work, but she was fobbed off, being told she couldn't call due to her son's privacy. Her intervention was badly needed, however, as David didn't notice what was going on anymore; he had lost himself totally. He told his psychiatrist that he was very suicidal, but the psychiatrist said he needed to wait longer, so he believed in that.

After five months, he got a new psychiatrist who told him to quit sertraline since it obviously didn't work, cold turkey, in just two weeks. At first, he got a one-day long mania and called his mother, telling her he hadn't felt so awesome before. After that, he got into horrible withdrawal where he couldn't sleep. .

This went on for months and didn't get better, and the emptiness took over more and more. In the first few months of withdrawal, he told his psychiatrist how he felt, but she didn't believe him. She told him it was not due to the drug, as it was out of his system. She said it was probably his obsessive, compulsive disorder that created all the problems.

David wrote in a suicide note that, "You present them with a problem that is created by the treatment you got from them, and as a reaction, get blamed yourself."

His life had stopped. He couldn't get pleasure out of anything. Even easy entertainment like gaming, something he had always enjoyed, gave him nothing. Everything was grey. Although he didn't feel anything by meeting girls anymore, his zero libido and erection problems weren't even the worst part: "The total erasing of any pleasure in life, as if I have been stripped of all my dopamine, is life debilitating."

He realized he was doomed to be in this state forever and saw no other option than suicide. He was very rational about this decision. It was a kind of self-euthanasia, which his parents, both doctors, understood.

The blunting of his emotions was fatal. He didn't feel emotionally connected to people, wasn't able to feel joy in anything, not even music. His whole personality had been wiped out, and he felt he was already dead and not human anymore, an empty shell. The last year of his life he often said that he desperately wanted to live, but not as a kind of lobotomized zombie. David had never had any sleeping problems before he took sertraline, but the drug caused severe insomnia, which lasted till the day he killed himself.

David wanted his story to be told, as a warning to others. Both he and his mother had read my book,[38] but unfortunately, nothing could be done. If he had read it before he was put on sertraline, he might have refused to take the drug that killed him.

I have heard similar suicide stories, also from Denmark, where not only the sex life continued being destroyed, but where the patients also experienced severe anhedonia (inability to feel pleasure), flatness of emotions, memory problems and cognitive dysfunction, which some of them described as a chemical lobotomy. Patients who have come off psychosis pills have also sometimes complained of persistent sexual dysfunction, which might be related to the fact that they were unable to have any sex life while they were on the drugs, or that they were on depression pills simultaneously. There is still a lot we don't know about persistent harms after withdrawal.

If people who are not psychiatrists—for example, doctors who don't use psychiatric drugs, nurses, pharmacists, psychologists, social workers, and people with no formal education but who care about other people—took over the whole psychiatric enterprise tomorrow, it would mean tremendous progress.

There is no hope for psychiatry, which has degenerated so much, for so long, and is so harmful that it must be stopped. It is much better for us not to have a psychiatry at all than to have the one we have, or anything remotely similar.

We need to act collectively. This is our only chance. If one worker strikes because of inhumane working conditions, the boss doesn't care but just fires the worker. If everybody walks out, all of a sudden, he has to negotiate.

Everybody needs to "walk out" of psychiatry. This is why I have written this book. Human beings can accept almost anything, if they get used to it, no matter how horrible, unfair and unethical it is, and few will protest against a sick system because it could be uncomfortable or dangerous for them. This is why we have had slavery as an officially accepted norm for thousands of years. This is also how the Nazis came to power in Germany and kept it; people were too afraid to protest, as the Nazis murdered their enemies early on. Only two months after president Paul von Hindenburg made Adolf Hitler chancellor of Germany, on 30 January 1933, Hitler opened the first concentration camp in Dachau, outside München.

Can you name any influential politician, psychiatrist, psychologist, or patient advocate who has run a great personal risk by criticizing psychiatry? Perhaps you can name one or two. I can mention quite a few but that's because I am part of the resistance movement, like my grandfather was during the Nazi occupation of Denmark.[25] He survived despite being taken by the Gestapo and sentenced to a concentration camp. He saved many Jews; I want to save as many psychiatric patients as I can. History means a lot to me. If the psychiatrists had not forgotten *their* history, then perhaps we would have had a better psychiatry today, but they repeat the same mistakes they have repeated for over 150 years. When Margrethe Nielsen drew me into psychiatric research in 2007, it was with this proposal: "Is history repeating itself?" She compared benzodiazepines with SSRIs and showed that indeed it does (see Chapter 4).

I have the following suggestions.

1. Disband psychiatry as a medical specialty. In an evidence-based healthcare, we do not use interventions that do more harm than good, which is what psychiatry does. In the transition period, let psychologists who are against using psychiatric drugs be heads of psychiatric departments and give them the ultimate responsibility for the patients.

2. Psychiatrists should be re-educated so that they can function as psychologists. Those who are not willing to do this, should find themselves another job or retire early.

3. The focus should be on getting patients off psychiatric drugs, as they are harmful in the long run, and as the vast majority of

patients are on long-term therapy. Courses on drug withdrawal should be mandatory for everyone working with mental health patients, and all patients must be explained why they would likely get a better life without drugs.

4. Establish a 24-hour national helpline and associated website to provide advice and support for those adversely affected by prescribed drug dependency and withdrawal.

5. Provide tapering strips and other aids to help patients withdraw from their drugs at no cost for the patients.

6. Apologize. It means a lot for victims of abuse to get an apology. Governments must require of psychiatric associations that they apologize unconditionally to the general public about the immense harm they have inflicted on mental health patients by lying systematically to them, e.g. about the chemical imbalance, and by telling them that psychiatric drugs can protect against suicide or brain damage. If organizations are unwilling to do this, governments must do it for them and dissolve the organizations because they are harmful to society.

7. Stop using words such as psychiatry, psychiatrist, psychiatric disorder, psychiatric treatments, and psychiatric drugs, as they are stigmatizing and as patients and the general public associate them with bad outcomes.[40,43] Change the narrative and use terms such as mental health instead.

8. Leave mental health issues to psychologists and other caring professions, as what the patients need more than anything else is psychotherapy, empathy, caring, and other psychosocial interventions.

9. Discard psychiatric diagnosis systems like DSM-5 and ICD-11 entirely and focus on the patients' most important issues. Psychiatric diagnoses are so unspecific and unscientific that virtually the whole population could get at least one, and they don't fit with the issues patients have, but often lead to additional diagnoses and more harm for psychiatric "career" patients.

10. Make forced treatment unlawful. All treatment of mental health issues must be voluntary. Forced treatment does vastly more harm than good,[38,44,45] and is discriminating.

11. Make psychiatric drugs available only for use under strictly controlled circumstances:

 a) while patients are tapering off them; or

 b) in rare cases where it is impossible to taper off them because they have caused permanent brain damage, e.g. tardive dyskinesia; or

 c) in patients with alcoholic delirium and as sedatives under operations and other invasive procedures, e.g. colonoscopy, which can be extremely painful.

12. Make it unlawful to use drugs that are registered for non-psychiatric uses, e.g. antiepileptics, for mental health issues, as this is harmful.

13. No one working with mental health patients should be allowed to have financial conflicts of interest with any manufacturer of psychoactive drugs or other treatments, e.g. equipment for electroshock.

14. All rules about the need for a psychiatric diagnosis in order to get social benefits, or economic support to schools, must be removed, as they create an incentive for gluing psychiatric diagnoses to people instead of helping them, which would involve other interventions than drugs.

15. Everyone: Do what you can to change psychiatry's misleading narrative. Speak about depression pills, psychosis pills, speed on prescription, etc.

Videos of Lectures and Interviews

If you are interested in seeing some of the lectures I have held or interviews I have given, I have made it easy for you by listing those in English or with English subtitles that have been seen most often on YouTube as per March 2021 (in thousands):

Title (abbreviated)	Length	Views	Link
Big pharma is organized crime	7:42	416	https://bit.ly/2XcHMAz
Deadly Medicines and Organised Crime	54:05	66	https://bit.ly/2JADhrF
Crimes in the drug industry and the lies in psychiatry	15:44	55	https://bit.ly/39JSD7L
Overdiagnosed & overmedicated	1:32:46	43	https://bit.ly/2yrxfHk
Psychiatry has gone astray	6:19	36	https://bit.ly/2V16HV5
Screening for breast and prostate cancer	7:52	26	https://bit.ly/2wizL28
Psychiatric drugs, few benefit, many are harmed	58:23	26	https://bit.ly/3dSgSUw
Death of a whistleblower and Cochrane's moral collapse	1:06:56	24	https://bit.ly/3aUfZsw
Psychiatric drugs, few benefit, many are harmed	49:17	23	https://bit.ly/2Xb3iWm
Discussion, Gøtzsche & Whitaker, psychiatric epidemic	45:46	23	https://bit.ly/347xumS
Forced psychiatric treatment must be abolished	1:50:06	20	https://bit.ly/2JFXv32
Psychiatric drugs do more harm than good	2:10:41	14	https://bit.ly/39FrdQw
Prescription drugs are the third leading cause of death	18:06	14	https://bit.ly/3dWp3z1
Survival of a whistleblower	49:42	11	https://bit.ly/3dWXZQc
On the wrong track, psychiatric epidemic	53:22	10	https://bit.ly/2wSLNQ8

Table 5-2: Videos of Lectures and Interviews

About the Author

Professor Peter C Gøtzsche graduated as a Master of Science in biology and chemistry in 1974 and as a physician 1984. He is a specialist in internal medicine; worked with clinical trials and regulatory affairs in the drug industry 1975-83, and at hospitals in Copenhagen 1984-95. With about 80 others, he co-founded the Cochrane Collaboration in 1993 (the founder is Sir Iain Chalmers), and established the Nordic Cochrane Centre the same year. He became professor of Clinical Research Design and Analysis in 2010 at the University of Copenhagen and has been a member of the Cochrane Governing Board twice. He now works freelance. Became visiting Professor, Institute of Health & Society, Newcastle University in 2019. Founded the Institute for Scientific Freedom in 2019.

Gøtzsche has published more than 75 papers in "the big five" (*BMJ, Lancet, JAMA, Annals of Internal Medicine* and *New England Journal of Medicine*) and his scientific works have been cited over 150,000 times. His most recent books are:

- *Vaccines: truth, lies and controversy* (2020).

- *Survival in an overmedicated world: look up the evidence yourself* (2019).

- *Death of a whistleblower and Cochrane's moral collapse* (2019).

- *Deadly psychiatry and organised denial* (2015).

- *Deadly medicines and organised crime: How big pharma has corrupted health care* (2013) (Winner, British Medical Association's Annual Book Award in the category Basis of Medicine in 2014).

- *Mammography screening: truth, lies and controversy* (2012) (Winner of the Prescrire Prize 2012).

- *Rational diagnosis and treatment: evidence-based clinical decision-making* (2007).

Five of these books have appeared in multiple languages, see deadlymedicines.dk.

Gøtzsche has given numerous interviews, one of which, about organised crime in the drug industry, has been seen over 400,000 times on YouTube: https://www.youtube.com/watch?v=dozpAshvtsA. Gøtzsche was in *The Daily Show* in New York on 16 Sept 2014 where he played the role of Deep Throat revealing secrets about Big Pharma. A documentary film about his reform work in psychiatry, Diagnosing Psychiatry https://diagnosingpsychiatry.com/filmen/ appeared in 2017.

Gøtzsche has an interest in statistics and research methodology. He has co-authored the following guidelines for good reporting of research:

- CONSORT for randomized trials (www.consort-statement.org),

- STROBE for observational studies (www.strobe-statement.org),

- PRISMA for systematic reviews and meta-analyses (www.prisma-statement.org), and

- SPIRIT for trial protocols (www.spirit-statement.org).

Gøtzsche is Protector for the Hearing Voices Network in Denmark.

Websites: scientificfreedom.dk and deadlymedicines.dk

Twitter: @PGtzsche1

References

Chapter 1. This Book Might Save Your Life

1. Gøtzsche PC. *Deadly psychiatry and organised denial.* Copenhagen: People's Press; 2015.

2. Jorm AF, Korten AE, Jacomb PA, et al. "Mental health literacy": a survey of the public's ability to recognise mental disorders and their beliefs about the effectiveness of treatment. *Med J Aus* 1997;166:182-6.

3. Priest RG, Vize C, Roberts A, et al. Lay people's attitudes to treatment of depression: results of opinion poll for Defeat Depression Campaign just before its launch. *BMJ* 1996;313:858-9.

4. Paykel ES, Hart D, Priest RG. Changes in public attitudes to depression during the Defeat Depression Campaign. *Br J Psychiatry* 1998;173:519-22.

5. Read J, Timimi S, Bracken P, Brown M, Gøtzsche P, Gordon P, et al. Why did official accounts of antidepressant withdrawal symptoms differ so much from research findings and patients' experiences? Unpublished manuscript.

6. Kessing L, Hansen HV, Demyttenaere K, et al. Depressive and bipolar disorders: patients' attitudes and beliefs towards depression and antidepressants. *Psychological Medicine* 2005;35:1205-13.

7. McHugh RK, Whitton SW, Peckham AD, Welge JA, Otto MW. Patient preference for psychological vs pharmacologic treatment of psychiatric disorders: a meta-analytic review. *J Clin Psychiatry* 2013;74:595-602.

8. Olfson M, Blanco C, Marcus SC. Treatment of adult depression in the United States. JAMA Intern Med 2016;176:1482-91.

9. Breggin P. The most dangerous thing you will ever do. Mad in America 2020; March 2. www.madinamerica.com/2020/03/dangerous-thing-psychiatrist/.

10. Gøtzsche PC. Psychiatry gone astray. 2014; Jan 21. https://davidhealy.org/psychiatry-gone-astray/.

11. Breggin PR. *Brain-disabling treatments in psychiatry: drugs, electroshock, and the psychopharmaceutical complex.* New York: Springer; 2008.

12. Breggin PR. Intoxication anosognosia: the spellbinding effect of psychiatric drugs. *Ethical Hum Psychol Psychiatry* 2006;8:201-15.

13. Gøtzsche P. Surviving psychiatry: a typical case of serious psychiatric drug harms. Mad in America 2020; Jan 7. www.madinamerica.com/2020/01/surviving-psychiatry-typical-case-serious-psychiatric-drug-harms/.

14. Bielefeldt AØ, Danborg PB, Gøtzsche PC. Precursors to suicidality and violence on antidepressants: systematic review of trials in adult healthy volunteers. *J R Soc Med* 2016;109:381-92.

15. Maund E, Guski LS, Gøtzsche PC. Considering benefits and harms of duloxetine for treatment of stress urinary incontinence: a meta-analysis of clinical study reports. *CMAJ* 2017;189:E194-203.

16. Hengartner MP, Plöderl M. Newer-generation antidepressants and suicide risk in randomized controlled trials: a re-analysis of the FDA database. *Psychother Psychosom* 2019;88:247-8.

17. Hengartner MP, Plöderl M. Reply to the Letter to the Editor: "Newer-Generation Antidepressants and Suicide Risk: Thoughts on Hengartner and Plöderl's Re-Analysis." Psychother Psychosom 2019;88:373-4.

18. FDA package insert for Effexor. Accessed 4 Jan 2020. https://www.accessdata.fda.gov/drugsatfda_docs/label/2008/020151s051lbl.pdf.

19. FDA package insert for Neurontin. Accessed 4 Jan 2020. https://www.accessdata.fda.gov/drugsatfda_docs/label/2017/020235s064_020882s047_021129s046lbl.pdf

20. Horowitz MA, Taylor D. Tapering of SSRI treatment to mitigate withdrawal symptoms. *Lancet Psychiatry* 2019;6:538-46.

21. Davidsen AS, Jürgens G, Nielsen RE. Farmakologisk behandling af unipolar depression hos voksne i almen praksis. *Rationel Farmakoterapi* 2019; Nov.

22. Gøtzsche PC. Survival in an overmedicated world: look up the evidence yourself. Copenhagen: People's Press; 2019.

23. Demasi M, Gøtzsche PC. Presentation of benefits and harms of antidepressants on websites: cross sectional study. *Int J Risk Saf Med* 2020;31:53-65.

24. Whitaker R. *Anatomy of an epidemic, 2nd edition*. New York: Broadway Paperbacks; 2015.

Chapter 2. Is Psychiatry Evidence-Based?

1. Whitaker R. *Mad in America: bad science, bad medicine, and the enduring mistreatment of the mentally ill*. Cambridge: Perseus Books Group; 2002.

2. Healy D. *Let them eat Prozac*. New York: New York University Press; 2004.

3. Whitaker R. *Anatomy of an epidemic, 2nd edition*. New York: Broadway Paperbacks; 2015.

4. Gøtzsche PC. *Deadly psychiatry and organised denial*. Copenhagen: People's Press; 2015.

5. Medawar C. The antidepressant web—marketing depression and making medicines work. *Int J Risk & Saf Med* 1997;10:75-126.

6. Caplan PJ. *They say you're crazy: how the world's most powerful psychiatrists decide who's normal*. Jackson: Da Capo Press; 1995.

7 Breggin PR. *Brain-disabling treatments in psychiatry: drugs, electroshock, and the psychopharmaceutical complex*. New York: Springer; 2008.

8. Kirsch I. *The Emperor's new drugs: exploding the antidepressant myth*. New York: Basic Books; 2009.

9. Moncrieff J. *The bitterest pills*. Basingstoke: Palgrave Macmillan; 2013.

10. Davies J, ed. *The sedated society*. London: Palgrave Macmillan; 2017.

11. McLaren N. *Anxiety, the inside story. How biological psychiatry got it wrong*. Ann Arbor: Future Psychiatry Press; 2018.

12. Sharfstein S. Big Pharma and American psychiatry: The good, the bad and the ugly. *Psychiatric News* 2005;40:3.

13. Angermeyer MC, Holzinger A, Carta MG, et al. Biogenetic explanations and public acceptance of mental illness: systematic review of population studies. *Br J Psychiatry* 2011;199:367–72.

14. Read J, Haslam N, Magliano L. Prejudice, stigma and "schizophrenia:" the role of biogenetic ideology. In: *Models of Madness*. (John Read and JacquiDillon, eds.). London: Routledge, 2013.

15. Read J, Haslam N, Sayce L, et al. Prejudice and schizophrenia: a review of the "mental illness is an illness like any other" approach. *Acta Psychiatr Scand* 2006;114:303-18.

16. Kvaale EP, Haslam N, Gottdiener WH. The 'side effects' of medicalization: a meta-analytic review of how biogenetic explanations affect stigma. *Clin Psychol Rev* 2013;33:782–94.

17. Lebowitz MS, Ahn WK. Effects of biological explanations for mental disorders on clinicians' empathy. *Proc Natl Acad Sci USA* 2014;111:17786-90.

18. Davies J. *Cracked: why psychiatry is doing more harm than good.* London: Icon Books; 2013.

19. Kirk SA, Kutchins H. *The selling of DSM: the rhetoric of science in psychiatry.* New York: Aldine de Gruyter; 1992.

20. Williams JB, Gibbon M, First MB, et al. The Structured Clinical Interview for DSM-III-R (SCID). II. Multisite test-retest reliability. *Arch Gen Psychiatry* 1992;49:630-6.

21. Adult ADHD Self-Report Scale-V1.1 (ASRS-V1.1) Symptoms Checklist from *WHO Composite International Diagnostic Interview*; 2003.

22. Pedersen AT. En psykiatrisk diagnose hænger ved resten af livet. PsykiatriAvisen 2019; Jan 18. www.psykiatriavisen.dk/2019/ 01/18/ en-psykiatrisk-diagnose-haenger-ved-resten-af-livet/.

23. Frandsen P. Et anker af flamingo: Det, vi glemmer, gemmer vi i hjertet. Odense: Mellemgaard; 2019.

24. Pedersen AT. Diagnosing Psychiatry. https://vimeo.com/ondemand/ diagnosingpsychiatryen.

25. Breggin P. The most dangerous thing you will ever do. Mad in America 2020; March 2. www.madinamerica.com/2020/03/dangerous-thing-psychiatrist/.

26. Biederman J, Faraone S, Mick E, et al. Attention-deficit hyperactivity disorder and juvenile mania: an overlooked comorbidity? *J Am Acad Child Adolesc Psychiatry* 1996;35:997-1008.

27. Moreno C, Laje G, Blanco C, Jiang H, Schmidt AB, Olfson M. National trends in the outpatient diagnosis and treatment of bipolar disorder in youth. *Arch Gen Psychiatry* 2007;64:1032-9.

28. Gøtzsche PC. Psychopharmacology is not evidence-based medicine. In: James D (ed.). *The sedated society. The causes and harms of our psychiatric drug epidemic.* London: Palgrave Macmillan; 2017.

29. Varese F, Smeets F, Drukker M, Lieverse R, Lataster T, Viechtbauer W, et al. Childhood adversities increase the risk of psychosis: a meta-analysis of patient-control, prospective- and cross-sectional cohort studies. *Schizophr Bull* 2012;38:661-71.

30. Shevlin M, Houston JE, Dorahy MJ, Adamson G. Cumulative traumas and psychosis: an analysis of the national comorbidity survey and the British Psychiatric Morbidity Survey. *Schizophr Bull* 2008;34:193-9.

31. Kingdon D, Sharma T, Hart D and the Schizophrenia Subgroup of the Royal College of Psychiatrists' Changing Mind Campaign. What attitudes do psychiatrists hold towards people with mental illness? *Psychiatric Bulletin* 2004;28:401-6.

32. Demasi M, Gøtzsche PC. Presentation of benefits and harms of antidepressants on websites: cross sectional study. *Int J Risk Saf Med* 2020;31:53-65.

33. Kessing L, Hansen HV, Demyttenaere K, et al. Depressive and bipolar disorders: patients' attitudes and beliefs towards depression and antidepressants. *Psychological Medicine* 2005;35:1205-13.

34. Christensen AS. DR2 undersøger Danmark på piller. 2013; Mar 20. https://www.dr.dk/presse/dr2-undersoeger-danmark-paa-piller.

35. Ditzel EE. Psykiatri-professor om DR-historier: "Skræmmekampagne der kan koste liv." Journalisten 2013; Apr 11. https://journalisten.dk/psykiatri-professor-om-dr-historier-skraemmekampagne-der-kan-koste-liv/.

36. Gøtzsche PC. *Death of a whistleblower and Cochrane's moral collapse.* Copenhagen: People's Press; 2019.

37. Sterll B. Den psykiatriske epidemi. Psykolognyt 2013;20:8-11.

38. Gøtzsche PC. Psychiatry gone astray. 2014; Jan 21. https://davidhealy.org/psychiatry-gone-astray/.

39. Rasmussen LI. Industriens markedsføring er meget, meget effektiv. Den har fået lægerne til at tro på, at eksempelvis antidepressiva er effektive lægemidler. Det er de overhovedet ikke. Politiken 2015; Aug 30:PS 8-9.

40. Schultz J. Peter Gøtzsche melder psykiater til Lægeetisk Nævn. Dagens Medicin 2015; Oct 2. http://www.dagensmedicin.dk/nyheder/psykiatri/gotzsche-melder-psykiater-til-lageetisk-navn/.

41. Psykiatrifonden. Depression er en folkesygdom—især for kvinder. 2017; Jan 31. http://www.psykiatrifonden.dk/viden/gode-raad-og-temaer/depression/depression-er-en-folkesygdom.aspx.

42. Kessing LV. Depression, hvordan virker medicin. Patienthåndbogen 2015; July 5. https://www.sundhed.dk/borger/patienthaandbogen/psyke/sygdomme/laegemidler/depression-hvordan-virker-medicin/.

43. Videbech P. SSRI, antidepressivum. Patienthåndbogen 2015; July 23. https://www.sundhed.dk/borger/patienthaandbogen/psyke/sygdomme/laegemidler/ssri-antidepressivum/.

44. Scheuer SR. Studerende: Antidepressiv medicin er ikke løsningen på sjælelige problemer. *Kristeligt Dagblad* 2018; Mar 19.

45. Christensen DC. *Dear Luise: a story of power and powerlessness in Denmark's psychiatric care system.* Portland: Jorvik Press; 2012.

46. Angoa-Pérez M, Kane MJ, Briggs DI. et al. Mice genetically depleted of brain serotonin do not display a depression-like behavioral phenotype. *ACS Chem Neurosci* 2014;5:908-19.

47. Hindmarch I. Expanding the horizons of depression: beyond the monoamine hypothesis. Hum Psychopharmacol 2001;16:203-218.

48. Castrén E. Is mood chemistry? *Nat Rev Neurosci* 2005;6:241-6.

49. Gøtzsche PC, Dinnage O. What have antidepressants been tested for? A systematic review. *Int J Risk Saf Med* 2020;31:157-63.

50. Hyman SE, Nestler EJ. Initiation and adaptation: a paradigm for understanding psychotropic drug action. *Am J Psychiatry* 1996;153:151-62.

51. Gøtzsche PC. *Deadly medicines and organised crime: How big pharma has corrupted health care.* London: Radcliffe Publishing; 2013.

52. Moncrieff J, Cohen D. Do antidepressants cure or create abnormal brain states? *PLoS Med* 2006;3:e240.

53. Hamilton M. A rating scale for depression. *J Neurol Neurosurg Psychiat* 1960;23:56-62.

54. Gøtzsche PC. *Survival in an overmedicated world: look up the evidence yourself.* Copenhagen: People's Press; 2019.

55. Sharma T, Guski LS, Freund N, Gøtzsche PC. Suicidality and aggression during antidepressant treatment: systematic review and meta-analyses based on clinical study reports. *BMJ* 2016;352:i65.

56. Breggin P. *Psychiatric drug withdrawal: A guide for prescribers, therapists, patients and their families.* New York: Springer; 2012.

57. Davies J, Read J. A systematic review into the incidence, severity and duration of antidepressant withdrawal effects: Are guidelines evidence-based? *Addict Behav* 2019;97:111-21.

58. Danborg PB, Gøtzsche PC. Benefits and harms of antipsychotic drugs in drug-naïve patients with psychosis: A systematic review. *Int J Risk Saf Med* 2019;30:193-201.

59. Francey SM, O'Donoghue B, Nelson B, Graham J, Baldwin L, Yuen HP, et al. Psychosocial intervention with or without antipsychotic medication for first episode psychosis: a randomized noninferiority clinical trial. *Schizophr Bull Open* 2020; Mar 20. https://doi.org/10.1093/schizbullopen/sgaa015.

60. Bola J, Kao D, Soydan H, et al. Antipsychotic medication for early episode schizophrenia. *Cochrane Database Syst Rev* 2011;6:CD006374.

61. Demasi M. Cochrane – A sinking ship? *BMJ* 2018; 16 Sept. https://blogs.bmj.com/bmjebmspotlight/2018/09/16/cochrane-a-sinking-ship/.

62. Leucht S, Tardy M, Komossa K, et al. Antipsychotic drugs versus placebo for relapse prevention in schizophrenia: a systematic review and meta-analysis. *Lancet* 2012;379:2063-71.

63. Wunderink L, Nieboer RM, Wiersma D, et al. Recovery in remitted first-episode psychosis at 7 years of follow-up of an early dose reduction/discontinuation or maintenance treatment strategy: long-term follow-up of a 2-year randomized clinical trial. *JAMA Psychiatry* 2013;70:913-20.

64. Hui CLM, Honer WG, Lee EHM, Chang WC, Chan SKW, Chen ESM, et al. Long-term effects of discontinuation from antipsychotic maintenance following first-episode schizophrenia and related disorders: a 10 year follow-up of a randomised, double-blind trial. *Lancet Psychiatry* 2018;5:432-42.

65. Chen EY, Hui CL, Lam MM, Chiu CP, Law CW, Chung DW, et al. Maintenance treatment with quetiapine versus discontinuation after one year of treatment in patients with remitted first episode psychosis: randomised controlled trial. *BMJ* 2010;341:c4024.

66. Whitaker R. Lure of riches fuels testing. *Boston Globe* 1998; Nov 17.

67. Cole JO. Phenothiazine treatment in acute schizophrenia; effectiveness: the National Institute of Mental Health Psychopharmacology Service Center Collaborative Study Group. *Arch Gen Psychiatry* 1964;10:246-61.

68. Leucht S, Kane JM, Etschel E, et al. Linking the PANSS, BPRS, and CGI: clinical implications. *Neuropsychopharmacology* 2006;31:2318-25.

69. Khin NA, Chen YF, Yang Y, et al. Exploratory analyses of efficacy data from schizophrenia trials in support of new drug applications submitted to the US Food and Drug Administration. *J Clin Psychiatry* 2012;73:856–64.

70. Leucht S, Fennema H, Engel R, et al. What does the HAMD mean? *J Affect Disord* 2013;148:243-8.

71. Jakobsen JC, Katakam KK, Schou A, et al. Selective serotonin reuptake inhibitors versus placebo in patients with major depressive disorder. A systematic review with meta-analysis and Trial Sequential Analysis. *BMC Psychiatry* 2017;17:58.

72. Cipriani A, Zhou X, Del Giovane C, Hetrick SE, Qin B, Whittington C, et al. Comparative efficacy and tolerability of antidepressants for major depressive disorder in children and adolescents: a network meta-analysis. *Lancet* 2016;388:881-90.

73. Kirsch I, Deacon BJ, Huedo-Medina TB, et al. Initial severity and antidepressant benefits: A meta-analysis of data submitted to the Food and Drug Administration. *PLoS Med* 2008;5:e45.

74. Fournier JC, DeRubeis RJ, Hollon SD, et al. Antidepressant drug effects and depression severity: a patient-level meta-analysis. *JAMA* 2010;303:47-53.

75. Gøtzsche PC, Gøtzsche PK. Cognitive behavioural therapy halves the risk of repeated suicide attempts: systematic review. *J R Soc Med* 2017;110:404-10.

76. Moncrieff J, Wessely S, Hardy R. Active placebos versus antidepressants for depression. *Cochrane Database Syst Rev* 2004;1:CD003012.

77. Moncrieff J. *The myth of the chemical cure*. Basingstoke: Palgrave Macmillan; 2008.

78. Michelson D, Fava M, Amsterdam J, et al. Interruption of selective serotonin reuptake inhibitor treatment. Double-blind, placebo-controlled trial. *Br J Psychiatry* 2000;176:363-8.

79. Rosenbaum JF, Fava M, Hoog SL, et al. Selective serotonin reuptake inhibitor discontinuation syndrome: a randomised clinical trial. *Biol Psychiatry* 1998;44:77-87.

80. Breggin P. *Medication madness*. New York: St. Martin's Griffin; 2008.

81. Hughes S, Cohen D, Jaggi R. Differences in reporting serious adverse events in industry sponsored clinical trial registries and journal articles on antidepressant and antipsychotic drugs: a cross-sectional study. *BMJ Open* 2014;4:e005535.

82. Schneider LS, Dagerman KS, Insel P. Risk of death with atypical antipsychotic drug treatment for dementia: meta-analysis of randomized placebo-controlled trials. *JAMA* 2005;294:1934–43.

83. FDA. Alert for Healthcare Professionals: Risperidone (marketed as Risperdal). 2006; Sept https://www.fda.gov/Drugs/DrugSafety/PostmarketDrugSafetyInformationforPatientsandProviders/ucm152291.htm. Link inactive, as the issue has been described in the risperidone package insert:

https://www.accessdata.fda.
gov/drugsatfda_docs/label/2009/020272s056,020588s044,021346s03
3,021444s03lbl.pdf.

84. Koponen M, Taipale H, Lavikainen P, et al. Risk of mortality associated with antipsychotic monotherapy and polypharmacy among community-dwelling persons with Alzheimer's disease. J Alzheimers Dis 2017;56:107-18.

85. Gøtzsche PC. Psychiatry ignores an elephant in the room. Mad in America 2017; Sept 21. https://www.madinamerica.com/2017/09/psychiatry-ignores-elephant-room/.

86. Hegelstad WT, Larsen TK, Auestad B, et al. Long-term follow-up of the TIPS early detection in psychosis study: effects on 10-year outcome. *Am J Psychiatry* 2012;169:374-80.

87. Melle I, Olav Johannesen J, Haahr UH, et al. Causes and predictors of premature death in first-episode schizophrenia spectrum disorders. *World Psychiatry* 2017;16:217-8.

88. Chung DT, Ryan CJ, Hadzi-Pavlovic D, et al. Suicide rates after discharge from psychiatric facilities: a systematic review and meta-analysis. *JAMA Psychiatry* 2017;74:694-702.

89. Hjorthøj CR, Madsen T, Agerbo E et al. Risk of suicide according to level of psychiatric treatment: a nationwide nested case-control study. Soc *Psychiatry Psychiatr Epidemiol* 2014;49:1357–65.

90. Large MM, Ryan CJ. Disturbing findings about the risk of suicide and psychiatric hospitals. *Soc Psychiatry Psychiatr Epidemiol* 2014;49:1353–5.

91. Brown S. Excess mortality of schizophrenia. A meta-analysis. *Br J Psychiatry* 1997;171:502-8.

92. Wils RS, Gotfredsen DR, Hjorthøj C, et al. Antipsychotic medication and remission of psychotic symptoms 10 years after a first-episode psychosis. *Schizophr Res* 2017;182:42-8.

93. Forskningsrådet. *Tilgjengeliggjøring av forskningsdata.* 2017; Dec. ISBN 978-82-12-03653-6.

94. Gøtzsche PC. Does long term use of psychiatric drugs cause more harm than good? *BMJ* 2015;350:h2435.

95. Dold M, Li C, Tardy M, et al. Benzodiazepines for schizophrenia. *Cochrane Database Syst Rev* 2012;11:CD006391.

96. Coupland C, Dhiman P, Morriss R, et al. Antidepressant use and risk of adverse outcomes in older people: population based cohort study. *BMJ* 2011;343:d4551.

97. Bielefeldt AØ, Danborg PB, Gøtzsche PC. Precursors to suicidality and violence on antidepressants: systematic review of trials in adult healthy volunteers. *J R Soc Med* 2016;109:381-92.

98. Maund E, Guski LS, Gøtzsche PC. Considering benefits and harms of duloxetine for treatment of stress urinary incontinence: a meta-analysis of clinical study reports. *CMAJ* 2017;189:E194-203.

99. Hengartner MP, Plöderl M. Newer-generation antidepressants and suicide risk in randomized controlled trials: a re-analysis of the FDA database. Psychother Psychosom 2019;88:247-8.

100. Hengartner MP, Plöderl M. Reply to the Letter to the Editor: "Newer-Generation Antidepressants and Suicide Risk: Thoughts on Hengartner and Plöderl's Re-Analysis." *Psychother Psychosom* 2019;88:373-4.

101. Le Noury J, Nardo JM, Healy D, Jureidini J, Raven M, Tufanaru C, Abi-Jaoude E. Restoring Study 329: efficacy and harms of paroxetine and imipramine in treatment of major depression in adolescence. *BMJ* 2015;351:h4320.

102. Lars Kessing i Aftenshowet. *DR1* 2013; Apr 15.

103. Klein DF. The flawed basis for FDA post-marketing safety decisions: the example of antidepressants and children. *Neuropsychopharmacology* 2006;31:689–99.

104. Emslie GJ, Rush AJ, Weinberg WA, et al. Rintelmann J. A double-blind, randomized, placebo-controlled trial of fluoxetine in children and adolescents with depression. *Arch Gen Psychiatry* 1997;54:1031-7.

105. Eli Lilly and Company. Protocol B1Y-MC-X065. Clinical study main report: Fluoxetine versus placebo in the acute treatment of major depressive disorder in children and adolescents. 2000; Aug 8.

106. Eli Lilly and Company. Protocol B1Y-MC-HCJE. Clinical study report: Fluoxetine versus placebo in childhood/adolescent depression. 2000; 6 August.

107. Laughren TP. Overview for December 13 Meeting of Psychopharmacologic Drugs Advisory Committee (PDAC). 2006; Nov 16. www.fda.gov/ohrms/dockets/ac/06/briefing/2006-4272b1-01-FDA.pdf.

108. Vanderburg DG, Batzar E, Fogel I, et al. A pooled analysis of suicidality in double-blind, placebo-controlled studies of sertraline in adults. *J Clin Psychiatry* 2009;70:674-83.

109. Gunnell D, Saperia J, Ashby D. Selective serotonin reuptake inhibitors (SSRIs) and suicide in adults: meta-analysis of drug company data

from placebo controlled, randomised controlled trials submitted to the MHRA's safety review. *BMJ* 2005;330:385.

110. Fergusson D, Doucette S, Glass KC, et al. Association between suicide attempts and selective serotonin reuptake inhibitors: systematic review of randomised controlled trials. *BMJ* 2005;330:396.

111. FDA. Antidepressant use in children, adolescents, and adults. http://www.fda.gov/drugs/drugsafety/informationbydrugclass/ucm096273.htm.

112. Australian Government, Department of Health. The mental health of Australians. 2009 May. https://www1.health.gov.au/internet/publications/publishing.nsf/Content/mental-pubs-m-mhaust2-toc~mental-pubs-m-mhaust2-hig~mental-pubs-m-mhaust2-hig-sui.

113. Crowner ML, Douyon R, Convit A, Gaztanaga P, Volavka J, Bakall R. Akathisia and violence. *Psychopharmacol Bull* 1990;26:115-7.

114. Sharma T, Guski LS, Freund N, Meng DM, Gøtzsche PC. Drop-out rates in placebo-controlled trials of antidepressant drugs: A systematic review and meta-analysis based on clinical study reports. *Int J Risk Saf Med* 2019;30:217-32.

115. Paludan-Müller AS, Sharma T, Rasmussen K, Gøtzsche PC. Extensive selective reporting of quality of life in clinical study reports and publications of placebo-controlled trials of antidepressants. *Int J Risk Saf Med* 2021;32:87-99.

116. Montejo A, Llorca G, Izquierdo J, et al. Incidence of sexual dysfunction associated with antidepressant agents: a prospective multicenter study of 1022 outpatients. Spanish Working Group for the study of psychotropic-related sexual dysfunction. *J Clin Psychiatry* 2001;62 (suppl 3):10–21.

117. Healy D, Le Noury J, Mangin D. Enduring sexual dysfunction after treatment with antidepressants, 5α-reductase inhibitors and isotretinoin: 300 cases. *Int J Risk Saf Med* 2018;29:125-34.

118. Healy D, Le Noury J, Mangin D. Post-SSRI sexual dysfunction: Patient experi-ences of engagement with healthcare professionals. *Int J Risk Saf Med* 2019;30:167-78.

119. Healy D. Antidepressants and sexual dysfunction: a history. *J R Soc Med* 2020;113:133-5.

120. FDA package insert for Prozac. Accessed 14 March 2020. https://pi.lilly.com/us/prozac.pdf.

121. Medawar C, Hardon A. *Medicines out of control? Antidepressants and the conspiracy of goodwill*. Netherlands: Aksant Academic Publishers; 2004.

122. FDA package insert for Effexor. Accessed 4 Jan 2020. https://www.accessdata.fda.gov/drugsatfda_docs/label/2008/020151s051lbl.pdf.

123. FDA package insert for Lithobid. Accessed 12 March 2020. https://www.accessdata.fda.gov/drugsatfda_docs/label/2016/018027s059lbl.pdf.

124. Cipriani A, Hawton K, Stockton S, et al. Lithium in the prevention of suicide in mood disorders: updated systematic review and meta-analysis. *BMJ* 2013;346:f3646.

125. Börjesson J, Gøtzsche PC. Effect of lithium on suicide and mortality in mood disorders: A systematic review. *Int J Risk Saf Med* 2019;30:155-66.

126. FDA package insert for Neurontin. Accessed 4 Jan 2020. https://www.accessdata.fda.gov/drugsatfda_docs/label/2017/020235s064_020882s047_021129s046lbl.pdf.

127. Ghaemi SN. The failure to know what isn't known: negative publication bias with lamotrigine and a glimpse inside peer review. *Evid Based Ment Health* 2009;12:65-8.

128. Weingart SN, Wilson RM, Gibberd RW, et al. Epidemiology of medical error. *BMJ* 2000;320:774-7.

129. Starfield B. Is US health really the best in the world? *JAMA* 2000;284:483–5.

130. Lazarou J, Pomeranz BH, Corey PN. Incidence of adverse drug reactions in hospitalized patients: a meta-analysis of prospective studies. *JAMA* 1998;279:1200–5.

131. Ebbesen J, Buajordet I, Erikssen J, et al. Drug-related deaths in a department of internal medicine. *Arch Intern Med* 2001;161:2317–23.

132. Pirmohamed M, James S, Meakin S, et al. Adverse drug reactions as cause of admission to hospital: prospective analysis of 18 820 patients. *BMJ* 2004;329:15-9.

133. van der Hooft CS, Sturkenboom MC, van Grootheest K, et al. Adverse drug reaction-related hospitalisations: a nationwide study in The Netherlands. *Drug Saf* 2006;29:161-8.

134. Landrigan CP, Parry GJ, Bones CB, et al. Temporal trends in rates of patient harm resulting from medical care. *N Engl J Med* 2010;363:2124-34.

135. James JTA. A new, evidence-based estimate of patient harms associated with hospital care. *J Patient Saf* 2013;9:122-8.

136. Archibald K, Coleman R, Foster C. Open letter to UK Prime Minister David Cameron and Health Secretary Andrew Lansley on safety of medicines. *Lancet* 2011;377:1915.

137. Makary MA, Daniel M. Medical error—the third leading cause of death in the US. *BMJ* 2016;353:i2139.

138. Centers for Disease Control and Prevention. Leading causes of death. www.cdc. gov/nchs/fastats/lcod.htm.

139. WHO. Management of substance abuse. Amphetamine-like substances. Undated. Downloaded 14 March 2020. https://www.who.int/substance_abuse/facts/ATS/en/.

140. National Institute on Drug Abuse. What is the scope of methamphetamine misuse in the United States? 2019; Oct https://www.drugabuse.gov/publications/ research-reports/methamphetamine/what-scope-methamphetamine-misuse-in-united-states.

141. Moore TJ, Glenmullen J, Furberg CD. Prescription drugs associated with reports of violence towards others. *PLoS One* 2010;5:e15337.

142. Molina BS, Flory K, Hinshaw SP, et al. Delinquent behavior and emerging substance use in the MTA at 36 months: prevalence, course, and treatment effects. *J Am Acad Child Adolesc Psychiatry* 2007;46:1028-40.

143. The MTA Cooperative Group. A 14-month randomized clinical trial of treatment strategies for attention-deficit/hyperactivity disorder. *Arch Gen Psychiatry* 1999;56:1073-86.

144. Jensen PS, Arnold LE, Swanson JM, et al. 3-year follow-up of the NIMH MTA study. *J Am Acad Child Adolesc Psychiatry* 2007;46:989-1002.

145. Molina BS, Hinshaw SP, Swanson JM, et al. The MTA at 8 years: prospective follow-up of children treated for combined-type ADHD in a multisite study. *J Am Acad Child Adolesc Psychiatry* 2009;48:484-500.

146. Swanson JM, Arnold LE, Molina BSG, et al. Young adult outcomes in the follow-up of the multimodal treatment study of attention-deficit/hyperactivity disorder: symptom persistence, source discrepancy, and height suppression. *J Child Psychol Psychiatry* 2017;58:663-78.

147. Borcherding BG, Keysor CS, Rapoport JL, et al. Motor/vocal tics and compulsive behaviors on stimulant drugs: is there a common vulnerability? *Psychiatry Res* 1990;33:83-94.

148. Breggin PR. The rights af children and parents in regard to children receiving psychiatric diagnoses and drugs. *Children & Society* 2014;28:231-41.

149. Danborg PB, Simonsen AL, Gøtzsche PC. Impaired reproduction after exposure to ADHD drugs: Systematic review of animal studies. *Int J Risk Saf Med* 2017;29:107-24.

150. Cherland E, Fitzpatrick R. Psychotic side effects of psychostimulants: a 5-year review. *Can J Psychiatry* 1999;44:811-3.

151. Boesen K, Saiz LC, Erviti J, Storebø OJ, Gluud C, Gøtzsche PC, et al. The Cochrane Collaboration withdraws a review on methylphenidate for adults with attention deficit hyperactivity disorder. *Evid Based Med* 2017;22:143-7.

152. Storebø OJ, Ramstad E, Krogh HB, Nilausen TD, Skoog M, Holmskov M, et al. Methylphenidate for children and adolescents with attention deficit hyperactivity disorder (ADHD). *Cochrane Database Syst Rev* 2015;11:CD009885.

153. Boesen K, Paludan-Müller AS, Gøtzsche PC, Jørgensen KJ. Extended-release methylphenidate for attention deficit hyperactivity disorder (ADHD) in adults. *Cochrane Database Syst Rev* 2017;11:CD012857 (protocol; review in progress).

154. Wallach-Kildemoes H, Skovgaard AM, Thielen K, Pottegård A, Mortensen LH. Social adversity and regional differences in prescribing of ADHD medication for school-age children. *J Dev Behav Pediatr* 2015;36:330-41.

155. Morrow RL, Garland EJ, Wright JM, et al. Influence of relative age on diagnosis and treatment of attention-deficit/hyperactivity disorder in children. *CMAJ* 2012;184:755-62.

156. Santaguida P, MacQueen G, Keshavarz H, Levine M, Beyene J, Raina P. Treatment for depression after unsatisfactory response to SSRIs. Comparative effectiveness review No. 62. (Prepared by McMaster University Evidence-based Practice Center under Contract No. HHSA 290 2007 10060 I.) AHRQ Publication No.12-EHC050-EF. Rockville, MD: Agency for Healthcare Research and Quality; 2012: April. www.ahrq.gov/clinic/epcix.htm.

157. Rink L, Braun C, Bschor T, Henssler J, Franklin J, Baethge C. Dose increase versus unchanged continuation of antidepressants after initial antidepressant treatment failure in patients with major depressive disorder: a systematic review and meta-analysis of randomized, double-blind trials. *J Clin Psychiatry* 2018;79(3).

158. Samara MT, Klupp E, Helfer B, Rothe PH, Schneider-Thoma J, Leucht S. Increasing antipsychotic dose for non response in schizophrenia. *Cochrane Database Syst Rev* 2018;5:CD011883.

159. Miller M, Swanson SA, Azrael D, Pate V, Stürmer T. Antidepressant dose, age, and the risk of deliberate self-harm. *JAMA Intern Med* 2014;174:899-909.

160. Ho BC, Andreasen NC, Ziebell S, et al. Long-term antipsychotic treatment and brain volumes: a longitudinal study of first-episode schizophrenia. *Arch Gen Psychiatry* 2011;68:128-37.

161. Zipursky RB, Reilly TJ, Murray RM. The myth of schizophrenia as a progressive brain disease. *Schizophr Bull* 2013;39:1363-72.

162. Videbech P. Debatten om antidepressiv medicin—Virker det, og bliver man afhængig? *BestPractice Psykiatri/Neurologi* 2014; Maj:nr. 25.

163. Ownby RL, Crocco E, Acevedo A, et al. Depression and risk for Alzheimer disease: systematic review, meta-analysis, and meta-regression analysis. *Arch Gen Psychiatry* 2006;63:530-8.

164. Moraros J, Nwankwo C, Patten SB, Mousseau DD. The association of antidepressant drug usage with cognitive impairment or dementia, including Alzheimer disease: A systematic review and meta-analysis. *Depress Anxiety* 2017;34:217-26.

165. Coupland CAC, Hill T, Dening T, Morriss R, Moore M, Hippisley-Cox J. Anticholinergic drug exposure and the risk of dementia: a nested case-control study. *JAMA Intern Med* 2019; Jun 24.

166. Mojtabai R, Olfson M. National trends in psychotropic medication polypharmacy in office-based psychiatry. *Arch Gen Psychiatry* 2010;67:26-36.

167. Videos from International meeting: Psychiatric drugs do more harm than good. Copenhagen 2015; Sept 16. https://www.deadlymedicines.dk/wp-content/uploads/2014/10/International-meeting1.pdf

168. Gøtzsche PC. Long-term use of antipsychotics and antidepressants is not evidence-based. *Int J Risk Saf Med* 2020;31:37-42.

169. Belmaker RH, Wald D. Haloperidol in normals. *Br J Psychiatry* 1977;131:222-3.

170. Kroken RA, Kjelby E, Wentzel-Larsen T, Mellesdal LS, Jørgensen HA, Johnsen E. Time to discontinuation of antipsychotic drugs in a schizophrenia cohort: influence of current treatment strategies. *Ther Adv Psychopharmacol* 2014;4:228-39.

171. Nielsen M, Hansen EH, Gøtzsche PC. Dependence and withdrawal reactions to benzodiazepines and selective serotonin reuptake inhibitors. How did the health authorities react? *Int J Risk Saf Med* 2013;25:155-68.

172. Committee on the Review of Medicines. Systematic review of the benzodiazepines. Guidelines for data sheets on diazepam, chlordiazepoxide, medazepam, clorazepate, lorazepam, oxazepam, temazepam, triazolam, nitrazepam, and flurazepam. *Br Med J* 1980;280:910-2.

173. Gøtzsche PC. Long-term use of benzodiazepines, stimulants and lithium is not evidence-based. *Clin Neuropsychiatry* 2020;17:281-3.

174. Ilyas S, Moncrieff J. Trends in prescriptions and costs of drugs for mental disorders in England, 1998-2010. *Br J Psychiatry* 2012;200:393-8.

175. Nielsen M, Gøtzsche P. An analysis of psychotropic drug sales. Increasing sales of selective serotonin reuptake inhibitors are closely related to number of products. *Int J Risk Saf Med* 2011;23:125-32.

176. Nielsen M, Hansen EH, Gøtzsche PC. What is the difference between dependence and withdrawal reactions? A comparison of benzodiazepines and selective serotonin re-uptake inhibitors. *Addict* 2012;107:900-8.

177. Oswald I, Lewis SA, Dunleavy DL, Brezinova V, Briggs M. Drugs of dependence though not of abuse: fenfluramine and imipramine. *Br Med J* 1971;3:70-3.

178. Priest RG, Vize C, Roberts A, et al. Lay people's attitudes to treatment of depression: results of opinion poll for Defeat Depression Campaign just before its launch. *BMJ* 1996;313:858-9.

179. Read J, Timimi S, Bracken P, Brown M, Gøtzsche P, Gordon P, et al. Why did official accounts of antidepressant withdrawal symptoms differ so much from research findings and patients' experiences? Unpublished manuscript.

180. Public Health England. Dependence and withdrawal associated with some prescribed medications: an evidence Review. 2019; Sept. https://assets.publishing.service.gov.uk/government/uploads/system/uploads/attachment_data/file/829777/PHE_PMR_report.pdf.

181. Nutt DJ, Goodwin GM, Bhugra D, Fazel S, Lawrie S. Attacks on antidepressants: signs of deep-seated stigma? *Lancet Psychiatry* 2014;1:102-4.

182. Raven M. Depression and antidepressants in Australia and beyond: a critical public health analysis (PhD thesis). University of Wollongong, Australia; 2012. http://ro.uow.edu.au/theses/3686/.

183. Gøtzsche PC. Usage of depression pills almost halved among children in Denmark. Mad in America 2018; May 4. https://www.madinamerica.com/2018/05/usage-depression-pills-almost-halved-among-children-denmark/.

184. Chan A-W, Hróbjartsson A, Haahr MT, Gøtzsche PC, Altman DG. Empirical evidence for selective reporting of outcomes in randomized trials: comparison of protocols to published articles. *JAMA* 2004;291:2457-65.

185. Carney S, Geddes J. Electroconvulsive therapy. *BMJ* 2003;326:1343-4.

186. Read J, Bentall R. The effectiveness of electroconvulsive therapy: a literature review. *Epidemiol Psichiatr Soc* 2010 Oct-Dec;19:333-47.

187. Rose D, Fleischmann P, Wykes T, et al. Patients' perspectives on electro-convulsive therapy: systematic review. *BMJ* 2003;326:1363.

Chapter 3. Psychotherapy

1. Gøtzsche PC. *Deadly psychiatry and organised denial.* Copenhagen: People's Press; 2015.

2. Gøtzsche PC. Chemical or psychological psychotherapy? Mad in America 2017; Jan 29. https://www.madinamerica.com/2017/01/chemical-psychological-psychotherapy/.

3. Krupnick JL, Sotsky SM, Simmens S, et al. The role of the therapeutic alliance in psychotherapy and pharmacotherapy outcome: Findings in the National Institute of Mental Health Treatment of Depression Collaborative Research Program. *J Consult Clin Psychol* 1996;64:532–9.

4. Demyttenaere K, Donneau A-F, Albert A, et al. What is important in being cured from: Does discordance between physicians and patients matter? (2). *J Affect Disord* 2015;174:372–7.

5. Sørensen A, Gøtzsche. Antidepressant drugs are a type of maladaptive emotion regulation (submitted).

6. Spielmans GI, Berman MI, Usitalo AN. Psychotherapy versus second-generation antidepressants in the treatment of depression: a meta-analysis. *J Nerv Ment Dis* 2011;199:142–9.

7. Cuijpers P, Hollon SD, van Straten A, et al. Does cognitive behaviour therapy have an enduring effect that is superior to keeping patients on continuation pharmacotherapy? A meta-analysis. *BMJ Open* 2013;26;3(4).

8. Breggin PR. Intoxication anosognosia: the spellbinding effect of psychiatric drugs. *Ethical Hum Psychol Psychiatry* 2006;8:201–15.

9. Breggin PR. *Brain-disabling treatments in psychiatry: drugs, electroshock, and the psychopharmaceutical complex*. New York: Springer; 2008.

10. Gøtzsche PC, Gøtzsche PK. Cognitive behavioural therapy halves the risk of repeated suicide attempts: systematic review. *J R Soc Med* 2017;110:404-10.

11. Hawton K, Witt KG, Taylor Salisbury TL, et al. Psychosocial interventions for self-harm in adults. *Cochrane Database Syst Rev* 2016;5:CD012189.

12. Morrison AP, Turkington D, Pyle M, et al. Cognitive therapy for people with schizophrenia spectrum disorders not taking antipsychotic drugs: a single-blind randomised controlled trial. *Lancet* 2014;383:1395-403.

13. Seikkula J, AaltonenJ, Alakare B, et al. Five-year experience of first-episode nonaffective psychosis in open-dialogue approach: Treatment principles, follow-up outcomes, and two case studies. *Psychotherapy Research* 2006;16:214-28.

14. Svedberg B, Mesterton A, Cullberg J. First-episode non-affective psychosis in a total urban population: a 5-year follow-up. *Soc Psychiatry Psychiatr Epidemiol* 2001;36:332-7.

15. Harnisch H, Montgomery E. "What kept me going": A qualitative study of avoidant responses to war-related adversity and perpetration of violence by former forcibly recruited children and youth in the Acholi region of northern Uganda. *Soc Sci Med* 2017;188:100-8.

16. Nilsonne Å. Processen: möten, mediciner, beslut. Stockholm: *Natur & Kultur*; 2017.

Chapter 4. Withdrawing from Psychiatric Drugs

1. Gøtzsche PC. *Deadly medicines and organised crime: How big pharma has corrupted health care*. London: Radcliffe Publishing; 2013.

2. BBC. "My anti-depressant withdrawal was worse than depression." 2020 Mar 12. https://www.bbc.co.uk/programmes/p086fjk7.

3. Gøtzsche PC. Sundhedsstyrelsens råd om depressionspiller er farlige. *Politikens Kronik* 2010 Feb 6.

4. Horowitz MA, Taylor D. Tapering of SSRI treatment to mitigate withdrawal symptoms. *Lancet Psychiatry* 2019;6:538-46.

5. Gøtzsche PC. Prescription pills are Britain's third biggest killer: Side-effects of drugs taken for insomnia and anxiety kill thousands. Why do

doctors hand them out like Smarties? Daily Mail 2015; Sept 15. http://www.dailymail.co.uk/health/ article-3234334/Prescription-pills-Britain-s-biggest-killer-effects-drugs-taken-insomnia-anxiety-kill-thousands-doctors-hand-like-Smarties.html.

6. Gøtzsche PC. *Deadly psychiatry and organised denial.* Copenhagen: People's Press; 2015.

7. Gøtzsche PC. *Death of a whistleblower and Cochrane's moral collapse.* Copenhagen: People's Press; 2019.

8. Public Health England. Dependence and withdrawal associated with some prescribed medications: an evidence Review. 2019; Sept. https://assets.publishing.service.gov.uk/government/uploads/system/up loads/attachment_data/file/829777/PHE_PMR_report.pdf

9. Guy A, Davies J, Rizq R (eds.) Guidance for psychological therapists: Enabling conversations with clients taking or withdrawing from prescribed psychiatric drugs. London: *APPG for Prescribed Drug Dependence*; 2019 Dec.

10. Ho BC, Andreasen NC, Ziebell S, et al. Long-term antipsychotic treatment and brain volumes: a longitudinal study of first-episode schizophrenia. *Arch Gen Psychiatry* 2011;68:128-37.

11. Zipursky RB, Reilly TJ, Murray RM. The myth of schizophrenia as a progressive brain disease. Schizophr Bull 2013;39:1363-72.

12. Timimi S. Death of a whistleblower and Cochrane's moral collapse. Psychosis 2019; Oct 30. https://doi.org/10.1080/17522439.2019.1685584.

13. Gøtzsche PC, Sørensen A. The review on antidepressant withdrawal that Cochrane won't publish. Mad in America 2020; Feb 11. https://www.madinamerica.com/2020/02/review-cochrane-wont-publish/.

14. Cipriani A, Zhou X, Del Giovane C, Hetrick SE, Qin B, Whittington C, et al. Comparative efficacy and acceptability of 21 antidepressant drugs for the acute treatment of adults with major depressive disorder: a systematic review and network meta-analysis. *Lancet* 2018;391:1357-66.

15. Higgins JPT, Green S (eds.). Cochrane Handbook for Systematic Reviews of Interventions Version 5.1.0 [updated March 2011]. The Cochrane Collaboration, 2011. www.cochrane-handbook.org.

16. Gøtzsche PC. Rewarding the companies that cheated the most in antidepressant trials. Mad in America 2018; March 7. https://www.madinamerica.com/2018/03/rewarding-companies-cheated-most-antidepressant-trials/.

17. Munkholm K, Paludan-Müller AS, Boesen K. Considering the methodological limitations in the evidence base of antidepressants for depression: a reanalysis of a network meta-analysis. *BMJ Open* 2019;9:e024886.

18. Gøtzsche PC. Why we need a broad perspective on meta-analysis: It may be crucially important for patients. *BMJ* 2000;321:585-6.

19. Gøtzsche PC. Does long term use of psychiatric drugs cause more harm than good? *BMJ* 2015;350:h2435.

20. Davies J, Read J. A systematic review into the incidence, severity and duration of antidepressant withdrawal effects: Are guidelines evidence-based? *Addict Behav* 2019;97:111-21.

21. Groot PC, van Os J. How user knowledge of psychotropic drug withdrawal resulted in the development of person-specific tapering medication. *Ther Adv Psychopharmacol* 2020 Jul 10;10:2045125320932452.

22. www.survivingantidepressants.org. Surviving Antidepressants is a site for peer support, documentation, and education about withdrawal symptoms caused by depression pills, with more than 6,000 reports of patient experiences.

23. Inner Compass Initiative: The Withdrawal Project. https://withdrawal.theinnercompass.org. Resources for withdrawal from psychiatric drugs.

24. Hall W. Harm reduction guide to coming off psychiatric drugs. The Icarus Project and Freedom Center; 2012. www.theicarusproject.net/resources/publications/harm-reduction-guide-to-comingoff-psychiatric-drugs-and-withdrawal/.

25. Benzo buddies. Mutual-support environment for those who wish to withdraw from benzodiazepines. www.benzobuddies.org.

26. Recovery Road. Antidepressant & Benzodiazepine Withdrawal Support. www.recovery-road.org.

27. Ashton CH. Benzodiazepines: how they work and how to withdraw. Newcastle: University of Newcastle; 2011. www.benzo.org.uk/manual/.

28. Toft B, Gøtzsche PC. Psykofarmakaepidemien kan bekæmpes. Information 2017; Apr 3. https://www.information.dk/debat/2017/04/psykofarmakaepidemien-kan-bekaempes.

29. Gøtzsche PC. *Survival in an overmedicated world: look up the evidence yourself*. Copenhagen: People's Press; 2019.

30. McLaren N. *Anxiety, the inside story. How biological psychiatry got it wrong.* Ann Arbor: Future Psychiatry Press; 2018.

31. Christensen DC. *Dear Luise: a story of power and powerlessness in Denmark's psychiatric care system.* Portland: Jorvik Press; 2012.

32. Ostrow L, Jessell L, Hurd M, Darrow SM, Cohen D. Discontinuing psychiatric medications: a survey of long-term users. *Psychiatr Serv* 2017;68:1232-8.

33. Groot P, van Os J. Antidepressant tapering strips to help people come off medication more safely. *Psychosis* 2018;10:142-5.

34. Horowitz MA, Taylor D. Tapering of SSRI treatment to mitigate withdrawal symptoms. *Lancet Psychiatry* 2019;6:538-46.

35. Sørensen A, Rüdinger B, Gøtzsche PC, Toft BS. A practical guide to slow psychiatric drug withdrawal. Copenhagen 2020; Jan 4. https://www.deadly-medicines.dk/wp-content/uploads/A-practical-guide-to-drug-withdrawal.pdf.

36. Breggin P. *Psychiatric drug withdrawal: A guide for prescribers, therapists, patients and their families.* New York: Springer; 2012.

37. Simons P. Peer-support groups were right, guidelines were wrong: Dr. Mark Horowitz on tapering off antidepressants. Mad in America 2019; Mar 20. https://www.madinamerica.com/2019/03/peer-support-groups-right-official-guidelines-wrong-dr-mark-horowitz-tapering-off-antidepressants/.

38. Zinkler M, von Peter S. End coercion in mental health services—toward a system based on support only. *Laws* 2019;8:19.

39. Fiorillo A, De Rosa C, Del Vecchio V, Jurjanz L, Schnall K, Onchev G, et al. How to improve clinical practice on involuntary hospital admissions of psychiatric patients: suggestions from the EUNOMIA study. *European Psychiatry* 2011;26:201-7.

40. Scanlan JN. Interventions to reduce the use of seclusion and restraint in inpatient psychiatric settings: what we know so far, a review of the literature. *Int J Soc Psychiat* 2010;56:412–23.

41. Gøtzsche PC, Vinther S, Sørensen A. Forced medication in psychiatry: Patients' rights and the law not respected by Appeals Board in Denmark. *Clin Neuropsychiatry* 2019;16:229-33.

42. Gøtzsche PC, Sørensen A. Systematic violations of patients' rights and lack of safety: cohort of 30 patients forced to receive antipsychotics. *Ind J Med Ethics.* 2020;Oct-Dec;5(4) NS: 312-8. Free access.

43. Dold M, Li C, Tardy M, et al. Benzodiazepines for schizophrenia. *Cochrane Database Syst Rev* 2012;11:CD006391.

44. Frandsen P. *Et anker af flamingo: Det, vi glemmer, gemmer vi i hjertet.* Odense: Mellemgaard; 2019.

45. Breggin P. *Brain-disabling treatments in psychiatry: drugs, electroshock and the psychopharmaceutical complex.* New York: Springer; 2007.

46 What does akathisia and tardive dyskinesia look like? Videos of children and adults who have been permanently brain damaged by psychosis pills. Undated.
    https://www.deadlymedicines.dk/lectures/.

47. Moncrieff J. Antipsychotic maintenance treatment: time to rethink? *PLoS Med* 2015;12: e1001861.

48. Karon BP. All I know about Peter Breggin. In: The International Center for the Study of Psychiatry and Psychology. *The Conscience of Psychiatry. The reform work of Peter R. Breggin*, MD. New York: Lake Edge Press; 2009.

49. Gøtzsche PC. Forced drugging with antipsychotics is against the law: decision in Norway. Mad in America 2019; May 4. https://www.madinamerica.com/2019/05/forced-drugging-antipsychotics-against-law/.

50. Gottstein J. *The Zyprexa papers.* Anchorage: Jim Gottstein; 2020.

Chapter 5. Survival Kit for Young Psychiatrists in a Sick System

1. Drachmann H. Klinikchef må ikke længere arbejde som psykiater. *Politiken* 2013; Feb 1.

2. Hildebrandt S. Lars Søndergård mistænkes atter for at overmedicinere. *Dagens Medicin* 2015; Oct 23.

3. Hildebrandt S. "Det er monstrøse doser af medicin." *Dagens Medicin* 2015; Oct 23.

4. Schmidt M. Svar fra ledelsen i Psykiatrien Vest. *Dagens Medicin* 2015; Oct 23.

5. Hildebrandt S. Derfor er Lars Søndergårds supervisor sat under skærpet tilsyn. *Dagens Medicin* 2016; Mar 3.

6. Schizotypal Personality Disorder Test.
    https://illnessquiz.com/schizotypal-personality-disorder-test/.

7. Mayo Clinic. Schizotypal personality disorder.
    https://www.mayoclinic.org/dis-eases-conditions/schizotypal-personality-disorder/symptoms-causes/syc-20353919.

8. Börjesson J, Gøtzsche PC. Effect of lithium on suicide and mortality in mood disorders: A systematic review. *Int J Risk Saf Med* 2019;30:155-66.

9. Svensson P. Så stoppade GU-professor allmänhetens insyn i läke-medelsforskning. Göteborgs-posten 2018; Jan 20. http://www.gp.se/nyheter/g%C3%B6teborg/s%C3%A5-stoppade-gu-professor-allm%C3%A4nhetens-insyn-i-l%C3%A4ke-medelsforskning-1.5069930.

10. Sternbeck P. Brallorna nere på professorn Elias Eriksson. *Equal* 2018; Jan 16.

11. Riksdagens Ombudsman. Kritik mot Göteborgs universitet for hand-läggningen av en begäran om utlämnande av allmänna handlingar m.m. 2017; Dec 20:*Dnr* 7571-2016.

12. Gøtzsche PC, Gøtzsche PK. Cognitive behavioural therapy halves the risk of repeated suicide attempts: systematic review. *J R Soc Med* 2017;110:404-10.

13. Sveriges radio. Striden om de antidepressiva medlen. 2017; Aug 28. http://sverigesradio.se/sida/avsnitt/943828?programid=412.

14. Gøtzsche PC. National boards of health are unresponsive to children driven to suicide by depression pills. Mad in America 2020; Mar 15. https://www.madinamerica.com/2020/03/children-driven-suicide-depression-pills/.

15. Frankfurt HG. *On bullshit*. New Jersey: Princeton University Press; 2005.

16. Läkemedelsbehandling av depression, ångestsyndrom och tvångssyndrom hos barn och vuxna. *Läkemedelsverket* 2016; Dec 8.

17. Barczyk ZA, Rucklidge JJ, Eggleston M, Mulder RT. Psychotropic medication prescription rates and trends for New Zealand children and adolescents 2008-2016. *J Child Adolesc Psychopharmacol* 2020;30:87-96.

18. UNICEF Office of Research. Building the future: children and the sustainable development goals in rich countries. *Innocenti ReportCard* 14; 2017.

19. Hjelmeland H, Jaworski K, Knizek BL, Ian M. Problematic advice from suicide prevention experts. *Ethical Human Psychology and Psychiatry* 2018;20:79-85.

20. Whitaker R, Blumke D. Screening + drug treatment = increase in veteran suicides. Mad in America 2019; Nov 10. https://www.madinamerica.com/2019/11/ screening-drug-treatment-increase-veteran-suicides/.

21. Gøtzsche PC. *Deadly medicines and organised crime: How big pharma has corrupted health care.* London: Radcliffe Publishing; 2013.

22. Videos of talks presented at the inaugural symposium for the Institute for Scientific Freedom. 2019; Mar 9. https://www.youtube.com/playlist?list=PLoJ5D4KQ1G0Z_ZQo5AIIi uuspAKCnc49T.

23. Medawar C, Hardon A. *Medicines out of Control? Antidepressants and the conspiracy of goodwill.* Netherlands: Aksant Academic Publishers; 2004.

24. Stordrange IL. The happy pill. She survived 10 years of "torture" in psychiatry. 2017. https://www.youtube.com/watch?v=T4kVpNmYzBU&t=1s. Version with Norwegian subtitles: https://ingerlenestordrang.wixsite.com/lykkepillen.

25. Gøtzsche PC. *Survival in an overmedicated world: look up the evidence yourself.* Copenhagen: People's Press; 2019.

26. Hoel A. *Cause of death: unknown.* 2017; Mar 24. https://www.imdb.com/title /tt6151226/.

27. Jakobsen JC, Katakam KK, Schou A, et al. Selective serotonin reuptake inhibitors versus placebo in patients with major depressive disorder. A systematic review with meta-analysis and Trial Sequential Analysis. *BMC Psychiatry* 2017;17:58.

28. Gøtzsche PC. Antidepressiva skader mere end de gavner. *Dagens Medicin* 2017; Mar 15.

29. Gøtzsche P. The meeting was sponsored by merchants of death. Mad in America 2014; July 7. http://www.madinamerica.com/2014/07/meeting-sponsored-mer-chants-death/.

30. Pedersen AT. Diagnosing Psychiatry. https://vimeo.com/ondemand/diagnosingpsychiatryen.

31. Pedersen AT. Debat: Vi har ret til at undre os. *Journalisten* 2017; May 8.

32. Christensen AS. DR2 undersøger Danmark på piller. 2013; Mar 20. https://www.dr.dk/presse/dr2-undersoeger-danmark-paa-piller.

33. Ditzel EE. Psykiatri-professor om DR-historier: "Skræmmekampagne der kan koste liv." *Journalisten* 2013; Apr 11. https://journalisten.dk/psykiatri-professor-om-dr-historier-skraemmekampagne-der-kan-koste-liv/.

34. Gøtzsche PC. *Death of a whistleblower and Cochrane's moral collapse.* Copenhagen: People's Press; 2019.

35. Heilbuth PE. Pillens mørke skygge. DR1 2013; Apr 14.

36. Heilbuth PE. Dårlig presseetik, Politiken. *Politiken* 2013; Apr 19.

37. Thisted K. Jeg tager lykkepiller, ellers var jeg død! *Ekstra Bladet* 2015; Oct 24.

38. Gøtzsche PC. *Deadly psychiatry and organised denial*. Copenhagen: People's Press; 2015.

39. Spencer M. The Carter Center's guide for mental health journalism: don't question, follow the script. Mad in America 2020; Feb 23. https://www.madinamerica.com/2020/02/carter-center-guide-mental-health-journalism/.

40. Whitaker R. *Anatomy of an epidemic, 2nd edition*. New York: Broadway Paper-backs; 2015.

41. Gøtzsche PC. Psychiatry gone astray. 2014; Jan 21. https://davidhealy.org/psychi-atry-gone-astray/.

42. Gøtzsche PC. Unwarranted criticism of "Psychiatry cone astray." Mad in America 2014; Feb 20. https://www.madinamerica.com/2014/02/unwarranted-criticism-psychiatry-gone-astray/.

43. Jorm AF, Korten AE, Jacomb PA, et al. "Mental health literacy": a survey of the public's ability to recognise mental disorders and their beliefs about the effectiveness of treatment. *Med J Aus* 1997;166:182-6.

44. Gøtzsche PC, Vinther S, Sørensen A. Forced medication in psychiatry: Patients' rights and the law not respected by Appeals Board in Denmark. *Clin Neuropsychiatry* 2019;16:229-33.

45. Gøtzsche PC, Sørensen A. Systematic violations of patients' rights and lack of safety: cohort of 30 patients forced to receive antipsychotics. *Ind J Med Ethics*. 2020;Oct-Dec;5(4) NS: 312-8. Free access.

Index

Printed in the USA
CPSIA information can be obtained
at www.ICGtesting.com
LVHW010138080224
771247LV00015B/348